THE LAYMAN'S GUIDE
TO ACUPUNCTURE

8209

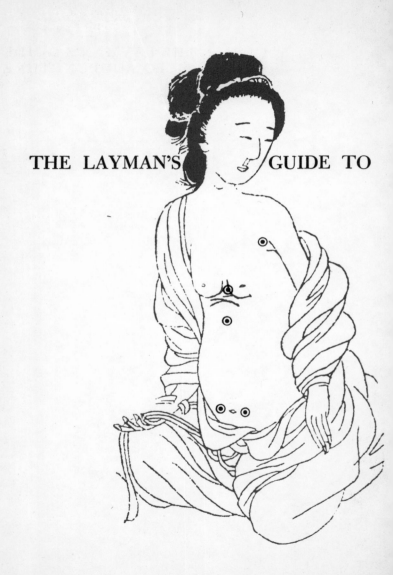

THE LAYMAN'S GUIDE TO

Yoshio Manaka, M.D.
and Ian A. Urquhart, Ph.D.

ACUPUNCTURE

with a foreword by Sally Reston

New York • WEATHERHILL • Tokyo

First Published 1972
Eighths Paperback Printed 1984

Published by John Weatherhill, Inc., of New York and
Tokyo, with editorial offices at 7-6-13 Roppongi,
Minato-ku, Tokyo 106. Protected by copyright under
terms of the International Copyright Union; all rights
reserved. Printed and first published in Japan.
LCC No. 72-78590   ISBN 0-8348-0107-8

To the ancient Chinese and Japanese who discovered and promulgated the laws of acupuncture;

To the modern practitioners of all nations who are willing to study, apply, and expand the ancients' knowledge;

To all patients and readers who are willing to investigate and possibly to accept a little-understood science;

To all who made this introductory study possible:

Our deep appreciation.

CONTENTS

LIST OF ILLUSTRATIONS

There are no miracles, only unknown laws.

SAINT AUGUSTINE

FOREWORD

YEARS AGO in one of those blinding English fogs, the morning London headline read: "FOG OVER CHANNEL—CONTINENT ISOLATED."

For twenty-two years there has been a political fog over the Pacific, separating in its shrouds the West and China. Sometimes, as the clouds lighten and new wonders are revealed, one asks who has been isolated from whom.

Nothing in the new look of China has surprised or fascinated the American people more than the picture of Chinese doctors using modern Western medical methods alongside ancient acupuncture. Originally skeptical, calling acupuncture "hypnosis" or even "quackupuncture," some American doctors now have had second thoughts and are, at least, suspending judgment. The National Institutes of Health have appointed experts to look into it. Dr. E. Gray Dimond, Provost of Health Sciences at the University of Missouri and colleague of Dr. Paul Dudley White in his Chinese medical investigations, has started studies of his own. Temple University Hospital in Philadelphia is using acupuncture for analgesia.

The Layman's Guide to Acupuncture—serious, well researched, and based on the authors' long experience—helps lift the old fog of ignorance. Surely, few subjects are so important as human suffering, and if the conclusions of this book can be extended and proved, the boon to mankind is clear.

Not a medical expert, I must be personal to be specific. Just before the President of the United States announced his dramatic visit to China, my husband and I were in Peking. Shortly after arrival, my husband was stricken with acute appendicitis, and underwent surgery and later acupuncture for relief from pain.

The Chinese doctors were intelligent, inventive, skillful, and kind. But the beginning of the adventure was not auspicious. As I helped my husband through the entrance to the Anti-Imperialism Hospital in Peking, we noticed a large gold-lettered slogan beside the door.

"The United States," it read, "and all its running dogs will be buried. There is certainly no escape for them. . . ."

It was a paradox, considering the peace, cleanliness, and compassion within, and I am glad to say that the slogan has now been taken down.

In some ways, we learned, the Chinese philosophy of medicine differs radically from that of the West. The Chinese use drugs sparingly, like to have their patients conscious even under major surgery, believing that postoperative recovery is more rapid, natural, and comfortable. With an area anesthetic, my husband was completely conscious during his operation, a Chinese diplomat from the Foreign Office standing by his head to interpret between patient and surgeon.

Two days later, the Chinese doctors, analyzing the pain that normally follows abdominal operations, proposed the use of acupuncture. Two needles were inserted slightly above the elbows and below the knees. For about fifteen minutes the acupuncturist shivered the needles intermittently while at the same time applying moxibustion.

Breaking in half a twelve-inch roll of paper filled with *ai* (*Artemisia vulgaris*), the acupuncturist lit both ends and twirled them, like two cigars, a little above the abdomen. As the smoke plumed upward, a nurse placed a paper with an inch-square hole at its center on the opposite side of the stomach, directing ultraviolet rays through the aperture. Whatever the scientific basis for the treatment (even the Chinese doctors readily admit they cannot explain—as is the case with aspirin—why acupuncture works), the result was relief.

Far more significant than this personal experience, however, is the new Chinese use of acupuncture as anesthesia. From a southern commune in Kwangtung Province where we saw two young "barefoot doctors" using acupuncture, to Dairen on the coast of Northeast China (Manchuria), to the surgical theaters of the large Shanghai hospitals, we followed the new discoveries in this ancient practice.

There was the fourteen-year-old boy, immobile for the last twelve from polio, who now, through combined therapy and acupuncture, walks with a cane. We watched the involuntary movement of his feet as acupuncture needles, carrying an electric charge of six volts, were inserted in his legs.

There was a twenty-six-year-old girl in Hun Shan Hospital in Shanghai who for twenty years had been fed through a tube. Tuberculosis in childhood had locked her jaw (ankylosis of the temporomandibular joint). Formerly given ether, it was three days after an operation before such patients could eat. Now with acupuncture the patient is conscious during surgery, sits up and eats ice cream before leaving the operating table.

In the Ninth Medical Hospital in Shanghai, they do three hundred tooth extractions a day with acupuncture for anesthesia. A needle is inserted in each *he ku* point, the "joined valley" between thumb and forefinger. Patients say they feel nothing more than a "mosquito bite" as the needles go in and nothing at all as the teeth come out. True, their faces did not wince, but mine did.

In the First Medical Hospital of Shanghai we watched an operation, started two hours earlier, for the removal of the right lung and one rib. A nurse sat by the patient's head, shaking a needle inserted at the *pi ju* point in the outer shoulder. While surgeons worked in a large cavity in the patient's back, we chatted with him.

In response to our questions, he told us his name was Chen Chun-kuo, he was twenty-four years old, had worked the last four years at the Yi Foodstuffs Company. From a stool at the other side of the operating table, while my husband conversed with the young man, I photographed his pulsating lung, clearly revealed in the surgical cavity. As we left the operating theater, Chen Chun-kuo ate orange sections from a spoon.

Was there some hidden hypnosis there we did not see? The Chinese deny it, saying that acupuncture anesthesia is used now on newborn babies and on animals.

Looking down from my hospital window into the narrow lanes of Peking, hearing the passing vegetable seller's flute, watching little boys with bamboo poles fishing up trees for the golden-winged locusts, I thought that China's wonders might surpass even the silks and spices of Marco Polo.

SALLY RESTON

AUTHORS' PREFACE

W HAT IS ACUPUNCTURE? Stated most simply, it is a therapy developed by the ancient Chinese that consists of stimulation of designated points on the skin by insertion of needles, application of heat, massage, or a combination of these. How and why this stimulation acts on the body is the subject of this book.

Following the example of pioneer researchers in both Europe and Asia, we will attempt to explain the principles and practice of acupuncture in terminology acceptable to modern medicine. So far, none of the answers proposed to the all-important questions of how and why has been entirely satisfactory or wholly demonstrable, and the doctor or layman interested in learning about acupuncture is likely to be discouraged by the massive technical dissertations dedicated to trying to answer these questions.

This has led us to attempt here to present the essentials of Chinese acupuncture in the most concise form possible. The reader will not find any of the elaborately reasoned deductions of Soulié de Morant, J. E. H. Niboyet, R. de la Fuye, A. Chamfrault, or others who have made major contributions to acupuncture studies in Europe. What he will find is a statement of principles whose application successfully alleviates many ills before which modern Western medicine remains disarmed.

It is not necessary to believe the ancient Chinese philosophy underlying acupuncture in order to practice it successfully but only to accept it as a working hypothesis until such time as it can be replaced by a more satisfactory theoretical framework. Should this book inspire one doctor with the desire to experiment with acupuncture, our work will not have been in vain. Should it help one person to understand the knowledge bequeathed us by the ancients to investigate and use, our labor will indeed have been worthwhile.

The Chinese names of the acupuncture meridians and points have been transliterated according to French spelling except where noted otherwise, because most of the important work on acupuncture in the West has been published in French, so that these spellings have become standard. Other Chinese words have been transliterated according to customary English romanization, as have Japanese terms.

THE LAYMAN'S GUIDE
TO ACUPUNCTURE

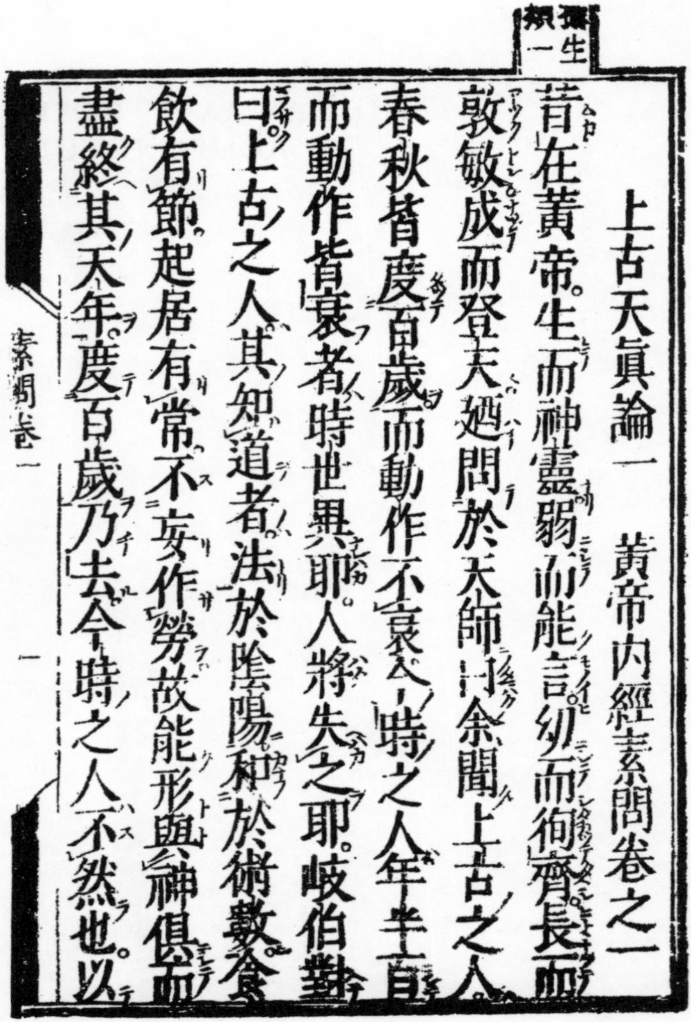

上古天眞論一　黄帝内經素問卷之一

昔在黄帝。生而神靈弱而能言幼而徇齊長而

敦敏成而登天廼問於天師曰余聞上古之人

春秋皆度百歲而動作不衰者一時之人年半百

而動作皆衰者時世異耶人將失之耶岐伯對

曰上古之人其知道者法於陰陽和於術數食

飲有節起居有常不妄作勞故能形與神俱而

盡終其天年度百歲乃去今時之人不然也以

素問卷一

一

1. The opening page of a Japanese edition of the Nei Ching.

1. AN INTRODUCTORY OVERVIEW

THE ORIGIN of Chinese medicine is lost in antiquity, though it is assumed to have developed from folk medicine. It has many aspects in common with other Oriental traditions, such as Indian herbal medicine and Persian medicine. The use of acupuncture, however, is unique to the Chinese branch of Oriental medicine.

The earliest known text on acupuncture is the *Nei Ching*, or Classic of Internal Medicine (fig. 1), traditionally ascribed to the legendary Yellow Emperor (Huang Ti, supposed to have lived 2697–2596 B.C.). Still extant, the *Nei Ching* remains the basic reference on the subject and is the foundation for all developments in acupuncture down to the present century.

In some manner the ancient Chinese became aware of an increased sensitivity of certain skin areas (called points) when a body organ or function was impaired. It was observed that in all patients the same skin areas became hypersensitive in the presence of a specific illness or organ dysfunction. Moreover, the sensitive areas varied consistently according to the organ function deviating from the norm. It was thus that some of the relationships among various internal organs and their functions were observed and established. These were defined and explained in terms of a complex philosophical hypothesis that attempted to relate all the phenomena observed.

Observation of hypersensitive skin areas in the presence of disease led to recognition of a series of such points existing concurrently during a specific illness that could be linked to organ dysfunction. These points were seen to follow a definite, invariable topographical pattern rather than to be scattered haphazardly over the body. Because they were well defined and constant in topographical presentation, these points could be used for diagnosing organ involvement in a variety of disorders. The line that could be drawn linking a series of points associated with a particular organ was called a meridian, and these meridians were identified with the various organs.

Acupuncture has a known history antedating Christianity by some two thousand years, so that over the course of centuries a long line of ancient practitioners, belonging to a people noted for meticulous visual observation, was able to establish the existence of a number of meridians and their relationships with various physiological functions. Some were related to specific internal organs, such as the heart, lungs, liver, and so on. Others were linked with organs not identified in Western medicine, such as the "heart constrictor" and the "triple heater." But it must be understood that the Chinese definition of organ is different from the Western one in certain important respects. To the Chinese an organ comprises not only an organic structure but also its entire functional system; organs are identified in terms of function rather than the other way around.

Fundamental to the concept of meridians in Chinese medicine is not only their function as imaginary lines linking a series of points on the skin that become sensitive in the presence of organic or functional disorders, but also their function as actual "energy pathways."

The theory of energy, or *ch'i*, set forth in the ancient Chinese texts is quite foreign to Western medical thought. According to the Chinese hypothesis, the body is endowed with a fixed energy quotient at birth. At the same time that this is depleted through the vicissitudes of daily living, it is augmented and transformed by energy obtained from food and air (food is considered to be a source of replenishment of depleted body energy rather than fuel to be metabolized by the body). Energy imbalance—its excess or insufficiency—is the root of illness; its absence is death.

This energy is considered to circulate throughout the body in a well-defined cycle, moving in a prescribed sequence from meridian to meridian and from organ to organ, flowing partly at the periphery and partly in the interior of the body. Like the Western concept of "nerve-energy potential" or the *prana* (life force) of Indian philosophy and medicine, *ch'i* is a dynamic force in constant flux.

This, briefly, is the body-energy concept in Chinese medicine, a hypothesis within whose framework the empirical therapy of acupuncture was developed.

Acupuncture was introduced to the West in the seventeenth century by Jesuit missionaries sent to Peking. Since that time several attempts have been made to promulgate this form of therapy in the Occident, with varying degrees of success. But not until the French Sinologist and diplomat Soulié de Morant published his voluminous writings on acupuncture in the 1940s did Western physicians have a sound basis for study and application of this ancient system of healing.

Under the impetus of de Morant's work, acupuncture associations and study groups were established in many Western countries, among them France, Italy, Britain, West Germany, Argentina, and the Socialist nations. These organizations are composed of physicians practicing a variety of specialties. (A list of the presidents of acupuncture organizations in over a score of nations is included as Appendix E.) In addition, many countries now support active research programs in the physiology and application of acupuncture, notably the USSR, the People's Republic of China, North and South Korea, and Japan.

Not only is acupuncture presently the focus of growing interest in the West, but it is undergoing a resurgence of serious study in the Orient, as well. In China, acupuncture is now an integral part of the nation's medical system, and an increasing number of press reports reach the West outlining some of its more startling applications there.

During the Long March of 1934–35, Mao Tse-tung's army lived and fought under the most primitive conditions and yet, using traditional Chinese medicine almost exclusively, managed to avoid epidemics and other serious illness. This led Mao to the pragmatic conclusion that acupuncture is effective and therefore should be used for the people.

It is unfortunate that the popular press often imputes to Chinese reports of acupuncture's efficacy a purely political motivation or otherwise assumes a derogatory attitude: the basic fact of the continuing popularity of acupuncture in the People's Republic of China is testimony of its effectiveness.

Japan officially established faculties of Western medicine at the university level in 1884, when Chinese medicine, practiced since the sixth century, was officially abandoned and proscribed. Nevertheless, it endured as an acceptable and effective method of treatment among the general populace and is now the object of much research at medical centers, hospitals, and universities. Today the Japanese public unhesitatingly uses the most advanced forms of Western medicine while retaining a close interest in and contact with this ancient method of healing that so often enhances the work done by Western-trained physicians and in innumerable cases solves problems that find no satisfactory solution in present Western medical knowledge.

The true field of acupuncture treatment is that of impaired body functions as opposed to actual lesions. In the case of a patient with diabetes, for example, if there is no actual tissue degeneration in the islets of Langerhans, acupuncture will be extremely effective. Even if lesions have formed and are well established, the pain, discomfort, and other symptoms caused by them are greatly relieved by acupuncture. But it is impossible to obtain complete and lasting relief of a functional problem that has an organic substratum. The basic organic disorder will always become discernible on application of acupuncture, and only temporary relief can be obtained, sometimes lasting only a few hours.

One of the primary functions of acupuncture is to affect directly the energy level, and therefore the functioning, of the internal organs by either stimulating or depressing their action. In many cases the liver can be activated when it is atonic or greatly calmed when in an irritated or congested condition. Tachycardia (rapid heart action) responds immediately to the correct application of acupuncture. Stomach and intestine action are notably modified in relation to function, and the action of the bladder and kidneys is also measurably increased or decreased through acupuncture. (In Chinese medicine, "action" may be considered to be the mechanical activity of an organ, while its "function" is of much wider scope. Inhalation and exhalation comprise the action of the lungs, for example, while their function includes the effects of respiration on the skin and on the metabolism in general.)

Some organs respond to acupuncture much more readily than others. The liver always responds extremely well, but the other internal organs are more difficult to control, most difficult being the kidneys. On the other hand, the spleen and gall bladder are both organs difficult to examine by Occidental methods, whereas their functions are ascertained and regulated with ease when examined by Chinese pulse diagnosis and treated by acupuncture.

As far as body energy, or *ch'i*, is concerned, acupuncture is indeed supreme in its effect. Pain of all kinds ceases immediately and often permanently, if there is no lesion, when acupuncture is properly applied to the appropriate meridian point or points. Contractures, no matter how chronic, are always quickly relieved. It is also possible to increase muscular strength by means of acupuncture because blood circulation is improved and hemoglobin production increased, leading to improved muscle tissue.

Statistics indicate success in 90 percent of cases involving pain, liver disorders, muscle contractures, and heart problems treated by acupuncture. Cases with bladder involvement show a 74 percent ratio of favorable response, and kidney problems a ratio of more than 60 percent. However, it is necessary to develop and expand the numerous statistical studies of acupuncture application and its results. Such studies should indicate whether failures are due to limitations in the method itself or to lack of knowledge in those applying it.

The area in which the efficacy of acupuncture has been most questioned is that of diseases attributed to microbe invasion, which have generally been considered beyond its scope. However, many such disorders do in fact respond with surprising speed. Many cases have been reported from China of cholera being relieved within a few hours by acupuncture.

The efficiency of the sense organs can also be enhanced through acupuncture. Reports of successful treatment of certain types of deafness and of eye problems are too numerous to be dismissed. Of particular interest is the successful treatment of color blindness, which will bar one from medical school and will, in Japan, deny one a driver's license. The mechanics of phenomena such as these are not easily explained in terms of present Western medical knowledge and are complex and difficult to explain even in the context of Chinese medicine; nevertheless, they do follow immutable physiological laws as defined by Chinese medicine.

One significant discovery that has been repeatedly verified by objective measurement is that acupuncture increases red-blood-cell (RBC) production. Researchers in both Japan and Europe have found that stimulation of a particular acupuncture point raises the RBC count of fully matured cells from a minus to a normal level within twenty-four hours. This level is maintained for four to six weeks, at which time the treatment is repeated; this continues until RBC production can be maintained at a normal level by the body itself as a result of treatment of the basic problem that caused the deficiency. The mechanics of this dramatic phenomenon are as yet imperfectly understood, but its implications are obvious.

The first question to be asked about acupuncture is whether it is worthwhile. If indeed it is successful in so many cases, a fact that can no longer be denied, then how and why is this so? The Chinese explain how and why acupuncture works by a philosophical hypothesis that in effect shifts the questions rather than answers them. They define the effects of acupuncture in terms of such concepts as the reflection of the universal energy of the macrocosm in the microcosm of man and the elements, elaborately relating all aspects of human physiology to natural phenomena. Obscure as such a hypothesis may initially appear, if the reader considers it carefully in the light of the results actually obtained through its application, he will find both the concepts and the procedures valid in the sense that they actually work; the principles can be verified through application.

The Chinese explanation is a pragmatic one, however exotic it may seem to those unfamiliar with Oriental thought; but Westerners seek a hypothesis that is not only empirically demonstrable but also intellectually satisfying within their own philosophical and scientific framework. Many researchers in both Europe and Asia have sought to formulate an alternative explanation of the facts that would be admissible to modern medical and scientific thought, in a terminology that would be intellectually acceptable. At present no altogether acceptable formulation exists. In view of this, we must recognize the tremendous value of the work being done in Western nations, particularly France, by physicians who, in striving to learn more about acupuncture, have courageously risked the opprobrium of their peers.

PART I

PRINCIPLES

2. THE CONCEPTS OF ENERGY AND YIN-YANG

THE CHINESE IDEOGRAM for "energy," pronounced *ch'i* (*ki* in Japanese), depicts the lid of a pot being raised by steam while on a fire. What is shown is not the steam but the force or energy of the steam. As with the falling apple of Newton, we see the effect (the lid being raised) but not the force causing the effect. This force, whether Newton's gravity or the Chinese *ch'i*, is extant though invisible.

The Chinese consider good health to be a state of energy balance within the human body; therefore they regard body tissues and structures primarily in relation to the energy activating them. There is in this a superficial similarity to the Western medical concept that an organ's activity is sustained by chemical and neurological impulses—in effect, energy.

But the Chinese view energy not only as the force maintaining bodily processes but as the primary component of all physiological activities. Furthermore, this energy varies not only quantitatively but qualitatively, manifesting in the polar forms of yin and yang energy.

Energy in its basic, undifferentiated state—as potential rather than active force—is termed *Tao*, the One underlying all phenomena. *Tao* is manifest in all things through the dynamic interaction of the two polar energy-forces called yin and yang, antagonistic yet complementary in action. As the *Nei Ching* states: "The universe is an oscillation of the forces of yin and yang and their changes."

There is no absolute yin or yang. Each exists relative to the other, and their relativity and inseparability are symbolized by the inclusion, in the Chinese yin-yang symbol, of a small portion of each within the other (fig. 2). Neither can exist without the other. This relativity of yin and yang and the dynamic tension of their interaction are the basis of thought and expression in Chinese philosophy, religion, literature, and art, as well as medicine.

We may think of yin and yang as the negative and positive poles, respectively, within a galvanic current flow; each is separate and distinct in expression, but both are part of the current. The current itself cannot exist without the bipolarity of its elements. The Chinese have extrapolated from this to consider the feminine as yin, the masculine as yang. Cold, dark, the passive, that which is deep or hidden are yin; heat, light, the active, that which is on the surface are yang. The earth and moon are associated with yin, the sky and sun with yang. Water is considered yin, while fire is considered yang. This dualism persists through all things: foods, attitudes, personal characteristics, and so on. At the same time, yin and yang are constantly interacting and changing, for one never exists in isolation from the other. In terms of medicine, this interaction is the basis of the energy pervading and activating the body, and imbalance in the relative amounts of yin and yang energy is seen as the root of all pathology.

This dynamic force of energy is constantly circulating within the body by means of the meridians; its movement in the body is a necessary condition for life. Energy is constant of itself but varies in manifestation. The Chinese use a simple example to illustrate this "changing sameness." A vertical plank has a top and a bottom; on reversing the ends of the plank the bottom becomes the top, and vice versa. The plank remains the same, but its parts have different names according to their positions relative to the center, and their properties vary according to their relative positions. The top has a greater energy potential than the bottom because of the force generated by falling. Likewise, the energy of the body is constant but shows different aspects according to the way it is used and the modifications it undergoes.

Detection of the presence of energy in the body has recently been the object of many studies and experiments, especially in Japan but also in other countries. In the *British Medical Journal* of February, 1937, Sir Thomas Lewis, in a paper entitled "An Unknown Nervous System," announced the discovery of a cutaneous nervous system "unsuspected at present," which is unrelated to the known sensory-nerve pathways and unconnected with the sympathetic nervous system: a system composed not of a network of nerves but of thin lines (as in fact the Chinese consider the meridians to be).

More recently, Dr. Kim Bon Hung of the University of Pyongyang in North Korea claimed to have discovered the meridians, so far considered to be imaginary lines of force, to be composed of a new type of actual histological tissue. But while his findings were apparently confirmed by one researcher in Japan, they have reportedly been negated by other investigators in both Japan and Europe.

As the above examples indicate, Western-oriented neurologists are concerned with the physical nerve pathways and their various pathological changes. In Chinese medicine, and Oriental medicine in general, however, there has been more concern with the quality or kind of impulse or charge passing along the energy pathways of the body (the meridians), which are now being viewed by some modern investigators of Chinese medicine as part of the autonomic nervous system.

In this context, the work of Dr. Nakatani in Osaka and of Professor Hyodo at the Osaka Medical University Pain Clinic, with their extensive neurometer examinations of patients, is of interest. Neurometer tests have established a correlation between changes in the electrical permeability of acupuncture

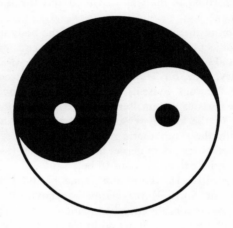

2. *The yin-yang symbol of China. There is no absolute yin or yang; this is why each is shown containing a portion of the other.*

points and syndromes clearly defined in Western medicine. Moreover, the acupuncture points registering this effect are associated with organs identical to those identified in connection with equivalent Western syndromes. Patients with whiplash injuries, for example, show a particular aberrant electrical pattern that has proved consistent in examinations of over one thousand cases. In short, the electrical permeability of the meridians shows definite, consistent changes in the presence of conditions equivalent to syndromes defined in Western medicine.

3. THE FIVE-ELEMENT THEORY
AND THE ORGANS

BASIC TO AN UNDERSTANDING of the Chinese five-element theory and to the concern with organic function over organic structure is recognition of the belief that the microcosm reflects the macrocosm: that "that which is below is similar to that on high."

Just as the antagonism of yin and yang generates energy within man, so are yin and yang manifest in varying proportions in all things, the proportions determining their forms and properties. In ancient times the Chinese established five basic elements that interact in a creative cycle to form all other substances (fig. 3). These elements are fire, water, earth, metal, and wood, with fire being most yang and water most yin. The other three elements comprise varying proportions of yin and yang and are of more or less equivalent valency, though having different properties. Each of the five elements is identified with a body organ, color, planet, compass direction, season, and so on, in a complicated set of concordances that serves the Chinese as a convenient mnemonic device (see chart in Appendix D). These concordances are used in diagnosis and treatment, in accordance with the principles of microcosm reflecting macrocosm and of function determining form.

Referring to the chart of five-element concordances, we can see from the following example how these are used in diagnosis.

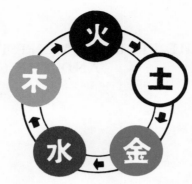

3. *The creative cycle of the five elements. Clockwise from top: fire, earth, metal, water, and wood.*

A patient with a "burned" body odor, a predilection for bitter-flavored food and drink, and a florid or "red" complexion, who sweats excessively, may well be subject to heart problems. It is worth repeating that to the Chinese a physiological organ, such as lungs, heart, or kidneys, includes not only its structure and physical location but also the entire system of functions associated with it. Thus, the organ of the heart includes not only the organic structure of that name and its mechanical pumping action but also the blood vessels and the energy of the blood circulation, as well as blood tissue. Likewise, the organ of the lungs includes both the function of respiration and its effects on the body and skin.

Thus the ancient anatomy charts of the Chinese do not show ignorance of physiology, as some have claimed, but illustrate their overriding concern with establishing the relationships between organs and functions, of which the meridians are an integral part. (It is this concern with function that led the Chinese to describe organs unknown in the West, such as the triple heater, or three metabolisms, and the heart constrictor, or master of the heart.)

To each of the five elements is assigned at least one yin and one yang organ, yin organs comprising those considered to have a predominantly internal function and yang organs those that

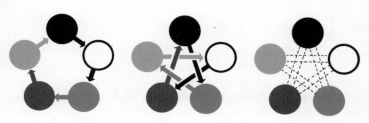

4. *The cycle of generation of the five elements (left): fire generates earth, earth generates metal, metal obtains water, water produces wood, and wood becomes fire. The cycle of destruction (center): water puts out fire, fire destroys metal, metal cuts down wood, wood covers earth, and earth absorbs water. Neutral relationships (right): water does not affect earth, earth does not affect wood, wood does not affect metal, metal does not affect fire, and fire does not affect water.*

function primarily in relationship to things outside the body. The yin organs include the liver, lungs, spleen-pancreas (the two were not differentiated by the ancient Chinese, though their importance and their various functions in digestion were recognized), kidneys, heart, and heart constrictor. The yang organs are the large intestine, small intestine, stomach, bladder, gall bladder (bile), and triple heater. They are identified with the five elements in the following manner:

fire: yin—heart, heart constrictor
          yang—small intestine, triple heater
earth: yin—spleen-pancreas
          yang—stomach
metal: yin—lungs
          yang—large intestine
water: yin—kidneys
          yang—bladder
wood: yin—liver
          yang—gall bladder

The five elements are generated and destroyed according to a law of cyclical interaction: fire produces earth, earth produces metal, metal finds water, water produces wood, and wood becomes fire. By substituting for each element a corresponding yin organ, for example, we see that the heart (fire) aids or reinforces the action of the spleen-pancreas (earth); the spleen-pancreas, the lungs (metal); the lungs, the kidneys (water); the kidneys, the liver (wood); and the liver, the heart. Conversely, just as fire melts metal, metal cuts down wood, wood covers earth, earth absorbs water, and water puts out fire, so the diseased or malfunctioning heart adversely affects the action of the lungs, the lungs affect the liver, the liver affects the spleen-pancreas, the spleen-pancreas affects the kidneys, and the kidneys affect the heart.

On the other hand, water is without effect on earth, earth does not affect wood, wood does not affect metal, metal does not affect fire, and fire does not affect water. Consequently, the kidneys do not affect the spleen-pancreas, the spleen-pancreas does not affect the liver, the liver does not affect the lungs, the lungs do not affect the heart, and the heart does not affect the kidneys (fig. 4).

4. ENERGY CIRCULATION: MERIDIANS AND POINTS

THE ENERGY GIVING LIFE to the body and activating each organ circulates in well-defined channels, called *ching* in Chinese and written with an ideogram that denotes the warp in weaving. In English they are called meridians, a word borrowed from geography that indicates an imaginary line joining a series of points. This is an apt term in that, like geographical meridians, the acupuncture meridians exist not as continuous lines but rather as series of points following linelike patterns.

There are twelve so-called "regular" meridians, one for each of the organs identified in the previous chapter, having identical branches on each bilateral half of the body. For example, the meridian of the heart is composed of a series of points beginning on the chest and running along the inside of the arm to the end of the little finger (fig. 9). These points on the skin, particularly those on the inside of the arm, exhibit a noticeably increased sensitivity when the heart is disturbed either organically or functionally.

Ten of the regular meridians are identified with structural organs also recognized in Western medicine: the lungs (L), large intestine (LI), stomach (S), spleen-pancreas (SP), heart (H), small intestine (SI), bladder (B), kidneys (K), liver (Li), and gall bladder (GB; figs. 5–14). The other two, those of the triple heater (TH) and heart constrictor (HC; figs. 15–16), are

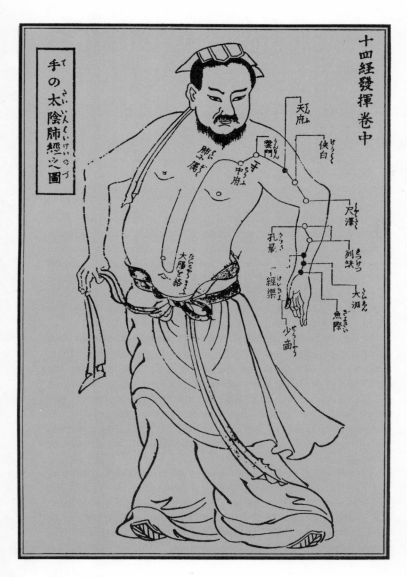

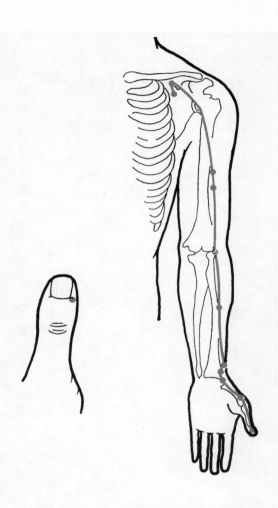

5. LUNG MERIDIAN. *This is a yin meridian with a descending flow of energy running from the chest to the hand. It has eleven bilateral points. Command points: wood, L 11; fire, L 10; earth, L 9; metal, L 8; water, L 5; origin, L 9; lo, L 7; gueki, L 6; alarm, L 1; iu, B 13.*

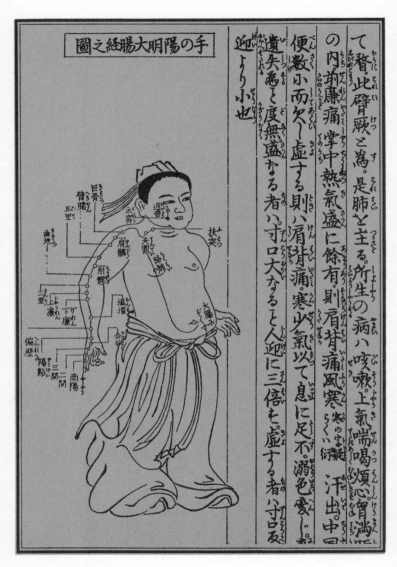

圖之經腸大明陽の手

て臂厥と爲す。是肺と主る。所生の病ハ咳嗽。上氣喘喝煩心胸滿肺　汗出中

の内前廉痛掌中熱氣盛に餘有。則肩背痛風寒

便數小而欠く虚する則ハ肩背痛。寒少氣以て息に足不。溺色變じ

遺失爲と度無盛たる者ハ寸口大なると人迎に三倍も虚する者ハ寸口反

迎より小也

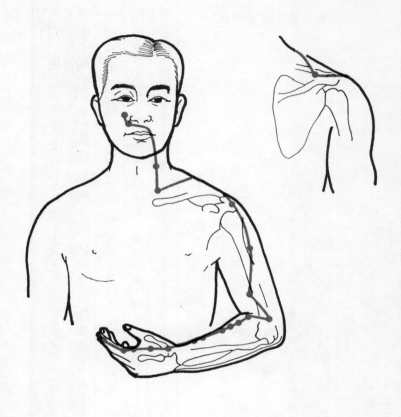

6. LARGE INTESTINE MERIDIAN. *This is a yang meridian with an ascending flow of energy running from the hand to the head. It has twenty bilateral points. Command points: wood, LI 3; fire, LI 5; earth, LI 11; metal, LI 1; water, LI 2; origin, LI 4; lo, LI 6; gueki, LI 7; alarm, S 25; iu, B 25.*

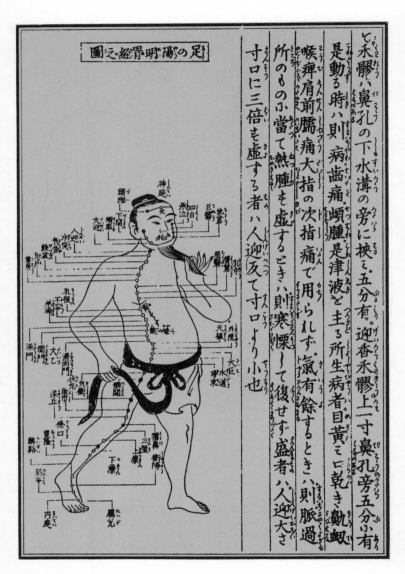

図之經の胃明陽の足

禾髎ハ、鼻孔の下水溝の旁に挾ミ.五分有。迎香禾髎上一寸鼻孔旁五分小有

是動る時ハ則チ病齒痛頰腫。是津液を主る所生病者目黃ミ口乾き齘齔

喉痺肩前臑痛大指の次指痛で用られず氣有餘するときハ則脈過

所のもの小當て熱腫を虛するときハ則寒慄して復せず盛者ハ人迎大さ

寸口に三倍を虛する者ハ人迎反て寸口より小也

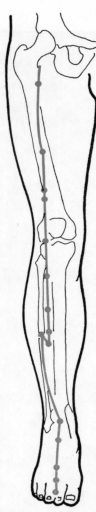

7. STOMACH MERIDIAN. *This is a yang meridian with a descending flow of energy running from the head to the foot. It has forty-five bilateral points. Command points: wood, S 43; fire, S 41; earth, S 36; metal, S 45; water, S 44; origin, S 42; lo, S 40; gueki, S 34; alarm, JM 12; iu, B 21.*

是動則病灑～然～而振寒善で伸。數欠顏黑病至則人火を悪水音と聞ば

惕然と而驚心動と欲獨戸牖を閉而處甚則高小上て歌衣を棄走賁嚮為

と欲腹脹是骭厥ぞ。是血主所生病ハ狂瘧温淫汗出衄口喝唇胗頸腫喉

痺大腹水腫膝臏腫痛脛氣街股伏兔骭外廉足の跗上を循皆痛中指用

そし氣盛なるとき、身以

前皆熱其胃に餘有則ハ

一穀を消し善飢溺の色黃

也氣不足なる則ハ身の

以前寒慄て胃中寒す

る則ハ脹滿を盛るゝ者ハ

人迎大なるを寸口小三倍

を虛なる者ハ人迎友て寸

口より小也

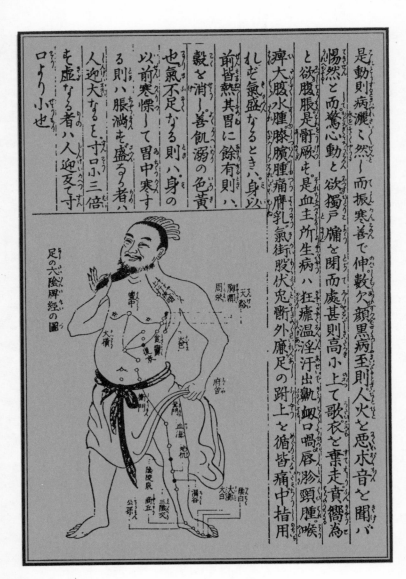

足の六陰脾經の圖

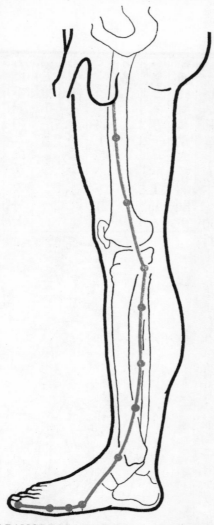

8. SPLEEN-PANCREAS MERIDIAN: *This is a yin meridian with an ascending flow of energy running from the foot to the chest. It has twenty-one bilateral points. Command points: wood, SP 1; fire, SP 2; earth, SP 3; metal, SP 5; water, SP 9; origin, SP 3; lo, SP 4; gueki, SP 8; alarm, Li 13; iu, B 20.*

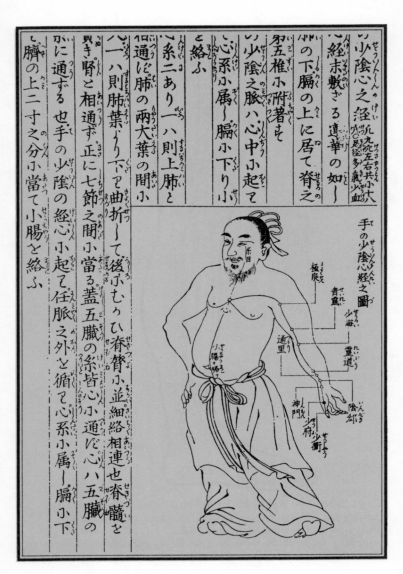

手の少陰心経之圖

○少陰心之経　脉九穴左右共小六
穴惠経悉多氣少血

○経末敷ざる遺華の如く

○の下膈の上に居て脊之

第五椎小附著そ

○少陰之脉ハ心中小起て

○心系小属し膈小下り小

と絡ふ

○系二あり一ハ上肺と

○通じ肺の兩大葉の間小

○一ハ則肺葉より下に曲折して後小むらひ脊簣小並細絡相連也脊髓を

○腎と相通ず正に七節之間小當る蓋五臟の糸皆心小通じ心ハ五臟の

がに通ずる也手の少陰の経心小起て任脈之外と循て心系小属し膈小下

し臍の上二寸之分小當て小腸と絡ふ

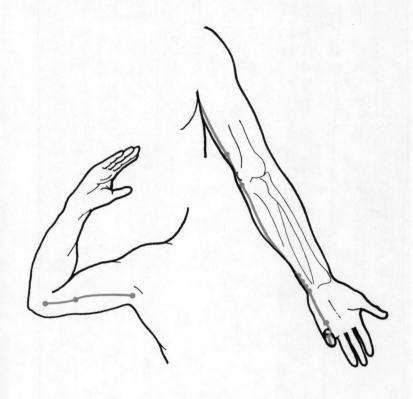

9. HEART MERIDIAN: *This is a yin meridian with a descending flow of energy running from the chest to the hand. It has nine bilateral points. Command points: wood, H 9; fire, H 8; earth, H 7; metal, H 4; water, H 3; origin, H 7; lo, H 5; gueki, H 6; alarm, JM 14; iu, B 15.*

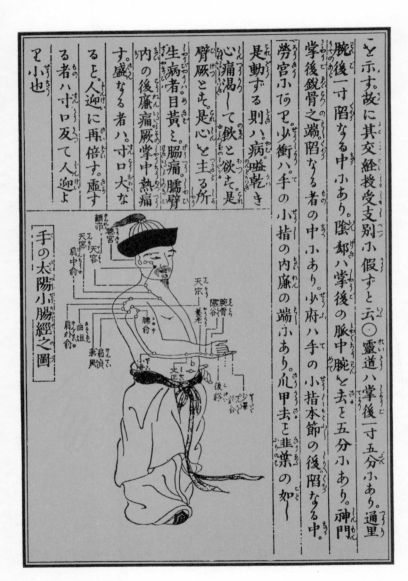

こと示す。故に其交經受支別小假すと云◯靈道八掌後一寸五分小あり。通里

腕後一寸陷なる中小あり。陰郄八掌後の脉中腕と去る五分小あり。神門

掌後鋭骨之端陷なる者の中小あり。少府八手の小指本節の後陷なる中。

勞宮小たゞ少衝八手の小指の内廉の端小あり。爪甲去る韮葉の如く

是動ずる則ハ病嗌乾き

心痛渇して飲と欲す。是

臂厥とも。是心と主る所

生病者目黄を脇痛臑臂

内の後廉痛厥掌中熱痛

す。盛なる者ハ寸口大な

ると人迎に再倍す。虚す

る者ハ寸口反て人迎よ

り小也

手の太陽小腸經之圖

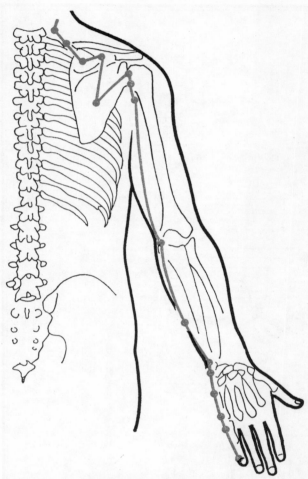

10. SMALL INTESTINE MERIDIAN. *This is a yang meridian with an ascending flow of energy running from the hand to the head. It has nineteen bilateral points. Command points: wood, SI 3; fire, SI 5; earth, SI 8; metal, SI 1; water, SI 2; origin, SI 4; lo, SI 7; gueki, SI 6; alarm, JM 4; iu, B 27.*

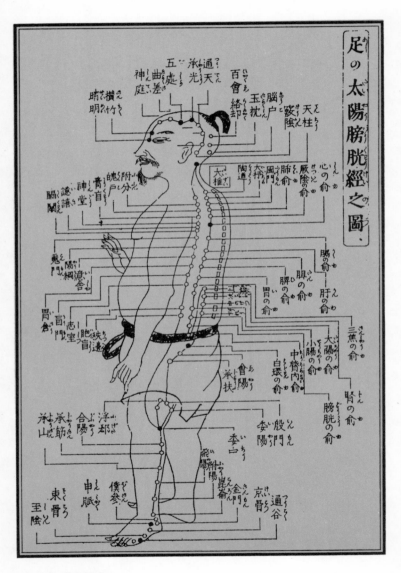

足の太陽膀胱經之圖、

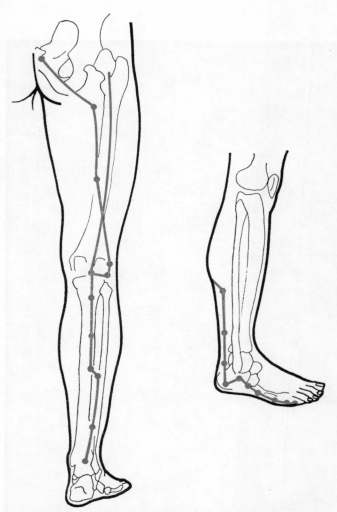

11. BLADDER MERIDIAN. *This is a yang meridian with a descending flow of energy running from the head to the foot. It has sixty-seven bilateral points. Command points: wood, B 65; fire, B 60; earth, B 54; metal, B 67; water, B 66; origin, B 64; lo, B 58; gueki, B 63; alarm, JM 3; iu, B 28.*

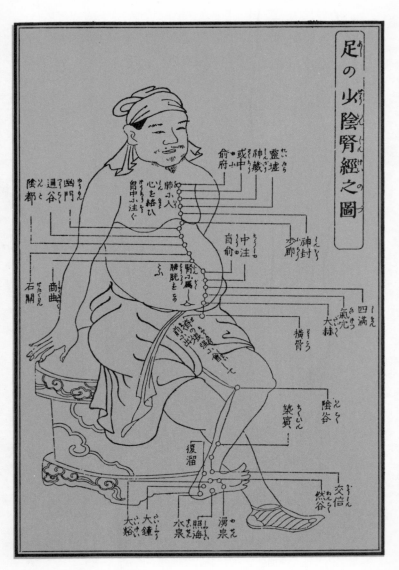

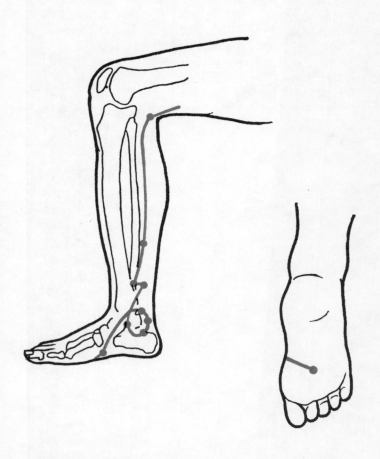

12. KIDNEY MERIDIAN. *This is a yin meridian with an ascending flow of energy running from the foot to the chest. It has twenty-seven bilateral points. Command points: wood, K 1; fire, K 2; earth, K 6; metal, K 7; water, K 10; origin, K 3; lo, K 4; gueki, K 5; alarm, GB 25; iu, B 23.*

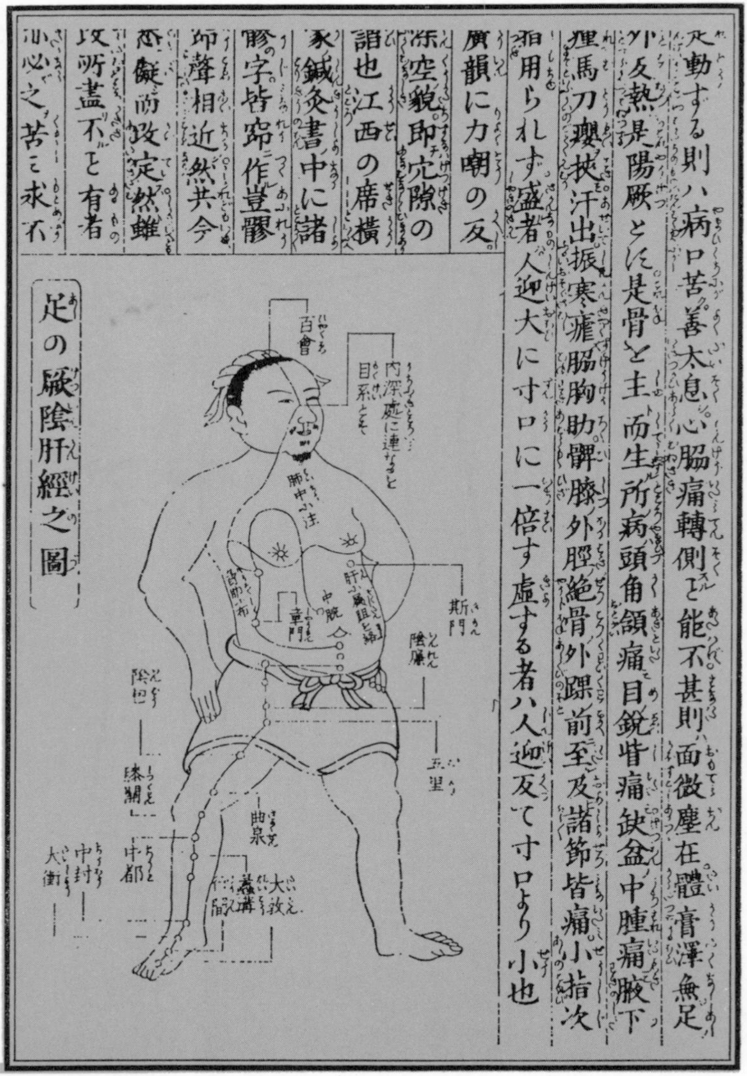

足動する則ハ病口苦ク善ク太息シ心脇痛轉側ニ能ヘス甚則ハ面微塵在體膏澤無足

ハ反シテ熱是陽厥とに是骨と主而生所病頭角頷痛目銳皆痛缺盆中腫痛腋下

狸馬刀瘻挾汗出振寒瘧脇胸肋髀膝外脛絶骨外踝前至及諸節皆痛小指次

用られす盛者人迎大に寸口に一倍す虚する者ハ人迎反て寸口より小也

廣韻に力嘲の反

漆空貌即宛隙の

諸也江西の席橫

永鍼灸書中に諸

膠字皆窊作豎髎

いぬ聲相近然今

應凝而玟定然蠶

攻所盡不と有者

小必之苦之求不

足の厥陰肝經之圖

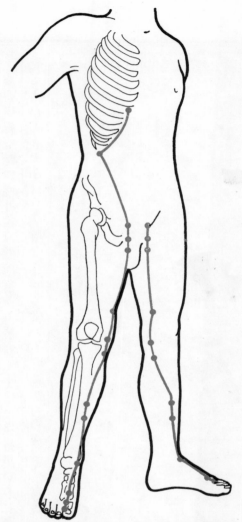

13. LIVER MERIDIAN. *This is a yin meridian with an ascending flow of energy running from the foot to the chest. It has fourteen bilateral points. Command points: wood, Li 1; fire, Li 2; earth, Li 3; metal, Li 4; water, Li 8; origin, Li 3; lo, Li 5; gueki, Li 6; alarm, Li 14; iu, B 18.*

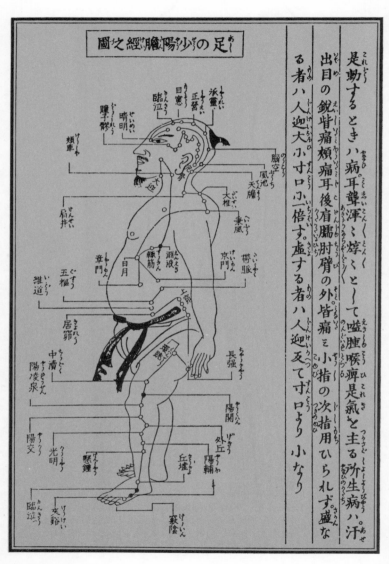

図之經膽陽少の足

承霊
正營
目窻
臨泣
瞳子髎
晴明
頰車
脳空
風池
天牖
大椎
眉井
秉風
章門
淵腋
輒筋
日月
京門
帯脈
五樞
維道
居髎
中瀆
陽陵泉
長強
陽關
外丘
陽輔
丘墟
陽交
光明
懸鐘
臨泣
侠谿
竅陰

是動するときハ病耳聾く渾く焞くとーて臨腫喉痺是氣と主る弥生病ハ汗出目の鋭眥痛頰痛耳後肩臑肘臂の外皆痛ミ小指の次指用ひられず盛なる者ハ人迎大小寸口ニ一倍す。虚する者ハ人迎反て寸口より小なり

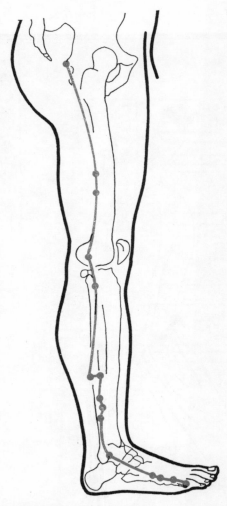

14. GALL BLADDER MERIDIAN. *This is a yang meridian having a descending flow of energy running from the head to the foot. It has forty-four bilateral points. Command points: wood, GB 41; fire, GB 38; earth, GB 34; metal, GB 44; water, GB 43; origin, GB 40; lo, GB 37; gueki, GB 36; alarm, GB 24; iu, B 19.*

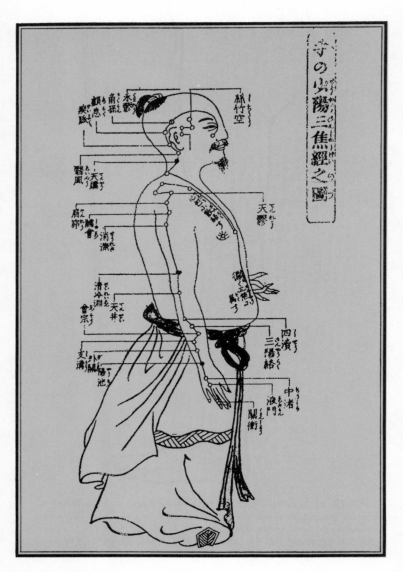

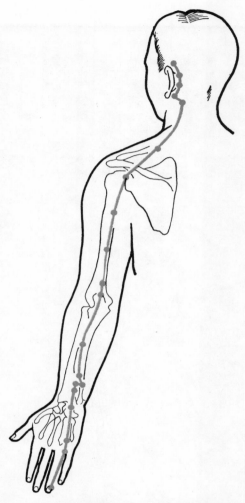

15. TRIPLE HEATER MERIDIAN. *Also called the three metabolisms, this is a yang meridian having an ascending flow of energy running from the hand to the head. It has twenty-three bilateral points. Command points: wood, TH 3; fire, TH 6; earth, TH 10; metal, TH 1; water, TH 2; origin, TH 4; lo, TH 5; gueki, TH 7; alarm, B 5; iu, B 22.*

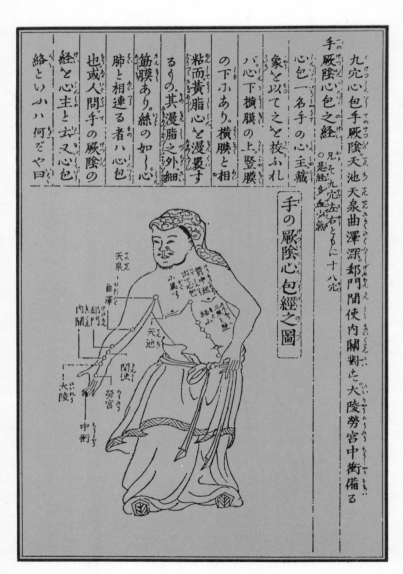

手の厥陰心包經之圖

九穴心包手厥陰。天池天泉曲澤深。郄門間使内關對。大陵勞宮中衝備る

○兄そ九穴左右ともに十八穴

手の厥陰心包之経

心包一名手の心主藏

象を以てこれを校ふれバ心下横膜の上堅膜

の下小あり。横膜と相粘而黄脂心と漫裏す

るの其漫脂之外細筋膜あり。絲の如く心

肺と相連る者ハ心包也或人間手の厥陰の

経と心主と云又心包絡といハ何ぞや曰

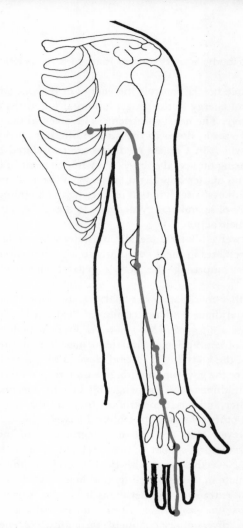

16. HEART CONSTRICTOR MERIDIAN. *Also called the master of the heart, this is a yin meridian with a descending flow of energy running from the chest to the hand. It has nine bilateral points. Command points: wood, HC 9; fire, HC 8; earth, HC 7; metal, HC 5; water, HC 3; origin, HC 7; lo, HC 6; gueki, HC 4; alarm, none identified; iu, B 14.*

related to body activity rather than to any specific organic body.

The triple heater controls the energy of respiration, the distribution of energy to the urogenital organs, and the energy of the sex drive. The heart constrictor is involved in the control of the blood vessels, down to the minute filtering portions of the kidneys, which in Chinese medicine are considered to have a direct bearing on sexual energy. (Any impairment in blood circulation, no matter how slight, adversely affects sexual energy, and the kidneys' vital function in filtering the blood means that the quality of sexual energy depends to a great extent on how efficient their action is.)

These twelve bilateral meridians are termed regular because energy circulates in them constantly in a specific direction and sequence, comprising the body's general energy-circulation system.

Two other meridians exist that are sometimes classified as regular meridians and sometimes as "extraordinary meridians." They are *jen-mô* (JM; *jenn-mo* in French spelling), or the meridian of conception, a unilateral meridian on the anterior midline of the body (fig. 17); and *tu-mô* (TM; *tou-mo* in French spelling), or the governor meridian, a unilateral meridian on the posterior midline of the body (fig. 18). Like the meridians of the triple heater and heart constrictor, they are free of any direct organ-structure relationship. Unlike the twelve bilateral meridians, however, they are not an integral part of the general energy-circulatory system but are related to it as secondary channels. Nevertheless, as with the bilateral meridians, energy does circulate in them constantly and in a prescribed direction.

Six true extraordinary meridians have also been identified: *yang-oe, yang-tsiao-mo, tae-mo, yin-oe, yin-tsiao-mo,* and *tchrong-mo.* These are "diversionary channels" through which energy flows only when pathological changes cause an excess of energy that the regular meridians cannot handle. The extraordinary meridians do not possess points exclusive to themselves but pass through certain points on the regular meridians (see the list of points of the extraordinary meridians on page 71), and energy does not flow through them in a consistent, invariable pattern. In addition, each possesses only one command point, called the master point, unlike the regular meridians, which have ten each (described later in this chapter).

A command point is a control point for energy flowing through a meridian and is therefore a major point in acupuncture treatment, though theoretically any point can be treated. It can be compared to the main lock of an irrigation system, which controls the entire flow of water in the main canal and its tributaries. The other points are like the locks of secondary canals, one or more of which may be opened to allow an extra flow of water to especially parched fields.

Jen-mô and *tu-mô* resemble the six extraordinary meridians in possessing only one such command point apiece. Having characteristics of both the regular and the extraordinary meridians, *jen-mô* and *tu-mô* are sometimes included in one group, sometimes in the other, depending on the properties under consideration.

The points on the meridians are not the only acupuncture points found on the skin. It has now been established that there are a number of effective acupuncture points outside the known meridians, called "extraordinary points beyond the meridians." So far they have not been associated with any specific organ or system, though the suggestion that they may be associated somehow with the endocrine system is being explored. Recent literature from the People's Republic of China has brought to light the efficacy of these additional points, and much research in this field is now under way in Japan.

The meridian points can be palpated by those with the proper training and are also electrically detectable (fig. 56). They invariably become sensitive in the presence of disturbed organ function. Several of the acupuncture points are known in Western medicine, such as McBurney's point on the abdomen, which is used in the diagnosis of appendicitis. Western medicine is also aware of some of the meridians, though they are not identified

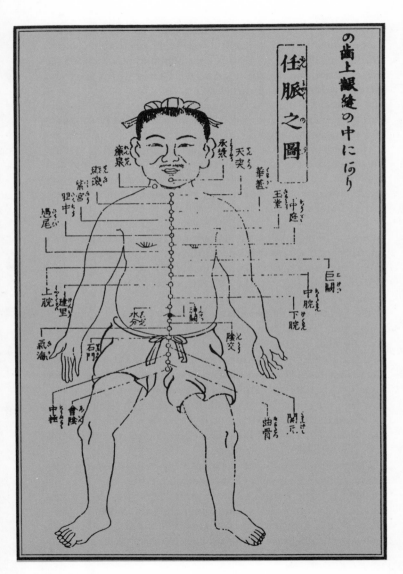

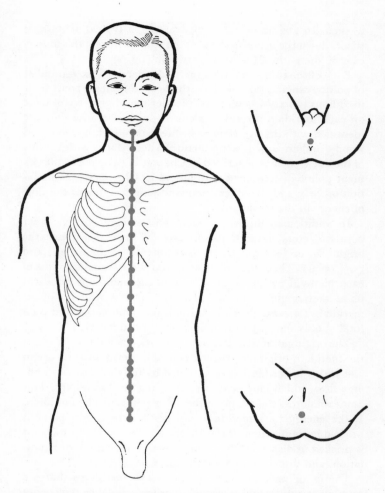

17. *JEN-MÔ* MERIDIAN. *Also called the meridian of conception, this meridian acts mainly on the yin energy. It is not an integral part of the general energy circulatory system but is related to it as a secondary channel. The energy flow is ascendant, running from the perineum to the chin. It carries twenty-four single points and is controlled by a single command point, L 7.*

as such. In angina pectoris, for example, a typical acute pain shoots down the inside of the arm to the little finger; this follows exactly the path of the heart meridian (fig. 9).

Each of the twelve bilateral meridians carries a fixed number of points, ranging from nine on the heart and heart constrictor meridians to sixty-seven on the bladder meridian. Five of these on each meridian are called element points, because they are identified with the five elements—fire, earth, metal, water, and wood—and are used in acupuncture in accordance with the law of the five elements, described in Chapter 3. (The use of the element points in treatment is discussed in Chapter 9). Stimulation of these and the other command points regulates the flow of energy in the meridians.

In addition to the five element points there are five other points of equal importance on each of these meridians: the origin; *lo*, or passage; *iu*, or assentiment; *mo*, or alarm; and *gueki* points. These ten points comprise the command points of each bilateral meridian. In several of the meridians the earth point and origin point are identical; this is why the heart meridian, for example, can have ten command points and yet a total of only nine separate points (see Appendix A).

The origin point is, as its name suggests, the point with which the meridian originates (which end of a meridian is its origin and which its terminus is determined by the direction of its energy flow, which may be either ascending or descending). This point reinforces the action of the other points on the meridian. If the energy in a meridian is depleted, the origin point is pricked in tonification. If the energy is in excess, the same point is pricked in dispersal (the techniques of tonification, or stimulation, and dispersal are described in Chapter 7).

The *lo,* or passage, point connects two meridians that are coupled at a pulse and is treated in order to balance the energy in such a pair of meridians (see Chapter 6 for a discussion of the pulses).

The *iu,* or assentiment, point is a diagnostic and treatment point for the visceral organs. The *iu* points of all the meridians are located on the bladder meridian (fig. 19).

The alarm, or *mo,* point becomes sensitive when the meridian on which it is located is disturbed and thus is a useful diagnostic indicator. The alarm point of a given meridian may or may not be located on its own meridian (fig. 20).

The *gueki* point usually becomes sensitive when its meridian is involved in acute rather than chronic illness. Unlike the other command points, the *gueki* point is located at some depth in the muscle and therefore is difficult to detect electrically.

The meridians having only one command point—*jen-mô, tu-mô,* and the six extraordinary meridians—can be divided into two groups of four yin and four yang meridians. The yin meridians include *jen-mô* (24 single points), *yin-oe* (3 single and 5 bilateral points), *yin-tsiao-mo* (1 single and 2 bilateral points), and *tchrong-mo* (1 single and 11 bilateral points). The yang meridians include *tu-mô* (27 single points), *yang-oe* (2 single and 15 bilateral points), *yang-tsiao-mo* (1 single and 11 bilateral points), and *tae-mo* (1 single and 3 bilateral points). The points of the six extraordinary meridians are listed below; those of *jen-mô* and *tu-mô* are shown in figures 17 and 18 respectively.

yin-oe: K 9, SP 13, SP 15, SP 16, Li 14, JM 22, JM 23, HC 6 (master point)

yin-tsiao-mo: K 6 (master point), K 8, B 1

tchrong-mo: K 11, K 12, K 13, K 14, K 15, K 16, K 17, K 18, K 19, K 20, K 21, SP 4 (master point)

yang-oe: B 63, GB 35, GB 24, SI 10, LI 14, GB 21, TH 15 (master point), GB 20, GB 19, GB 14, GB 13, GB 12, GB 11, GB 10, GB 9, TM 15, TM 14

yang-tsiao-mo: B 62 (master point), K 62, K 61, GB 38, GB 29, LI 15, LI 16, SI 10, S 7, S 6, S 4, K 1

tae-mo: GB 28, GB 27, GB 26, GB 41 (master point)

The master points on pairs of these meridians are coupled for treatment purposes, a point on the upper extremity of one me-

交經の支ハ。期門より肝小属處從別膽と貫き食實の外本經の裏と行上肺

に注下行て中焦至て中脘の分とさゝ挾む以て手の太陰に交る

是動する則病腰痛以俛仰為可不丈夫ハ癩疝婦人小腹腫甚き則嗌乾面塵色

脱是肝生所病胸滿嘔逆洞洩狐疝遺溺癃閉盛成者寸口大人迎小一倍虚す

者寸口反人迎從

小也○九で此十二經

病盛成則之瀉虚

為則之補熱為則

之疾寒為則之留

陷下為則之灸ー

盛ならば虚なら

ず經と以之と取

經穴の歌

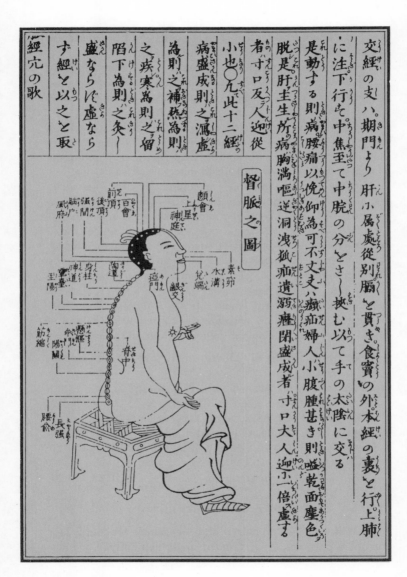

督脈之圖

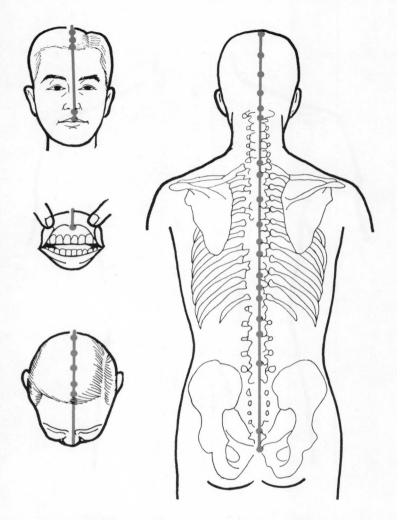

18. *TU-MÔ* MERIDIAN. *Also called the governor meridian, this meridian acts mainly on the yang energy. Like jen-mô, it is not part of the general energy circulatory system but is related to it as a secondary channel. The energy flow is ascendant, running from the coccyx to the upper gum. It carries twenty-seven single points and is controlled by a single command point, SI 3.*

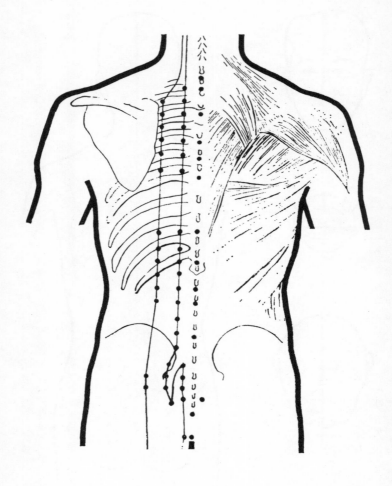

19. The iu, or assentiment, points. The iu point of each meridian lies on the bladder meridian: lung, B 13; large intestine, B 25; stomach, B 21; spleen-pancreas, B 20; heart, B 15; small intestine, B 27; bladder, B 28; kidney, B 23; liver, B 18; gall bladder, B 19; triple heater, B 22; heart constrictor, B 14.

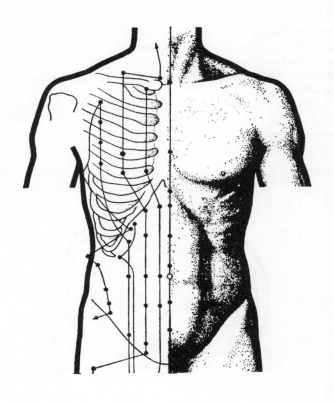

20. *The alarm, or* mo, *points. These may or may not be found on their own meridians. To some extent any point on a meridian can be considered an alarm point, its sensitivity indicating meridian disturbance. But the Chinese consider that the alarm points react most quickly, thus serving to indicate whether a diagnosis is correct or the treatment appropriate. Tenderness at these points is not a sign of visceral disease but an indication of meridian disturbance. The location of the alarm points may vary by a few millimeters from person to person. Following are the alarm points of the bilateral meridians: lung, L 1; large intestine, S 25; stomach, JM 12; spleen-pancreas, Li 13; heart, JM 14; small intestine, JM 4; bladder, JM 3; kidney, GB 25; liver, Li 14; gall bladder, GB 24; triple heater, B 5; heart constrictor, none identified.*

ridian being coupled with a point on the lower extremity of another, making four pairs of coupled master points: *jen-mô* (L 7) and *yin-tsiao-mo* (K 6); *yin-oe* (HC 6) and *tchrong-mo* (SP 4); *tu-mô* (SI 3) and *yang-tsiao-mo* (B 62); and *yang-oe* (TH 15) and *tae-mo* (GB 41).

These meridians can be treated at any of their points, but to treat the coupled master points effectively the two-metal-contact method (described in Chapter 11) or its equivalent, such as the insertion of two needles, is necessary.

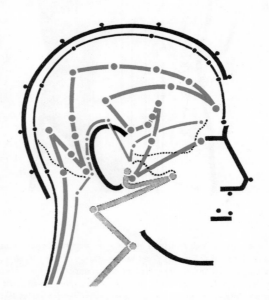

21. *Paths of the meridians on the face and head.* Tu-mô *points (large black dots)* 15, 16, 17, 18, 19, 20, 21, 22, 23, 24, 25, 26, 27. *Bladder points (small black dots)* 10, 9, 8, 7, 6, 5, 4, 3, 2. *Gall bladder points (large sepia dots)* 20, 19, 18, 17, 16, 15, 14, 13, 12, 11, 10, 9, 8, 7, 6, 5, 4, 3, 2, 1. *Triple heater points (small sepia dots)* 16, 17, 18, 19, 20, 21, 22, 23. *Small intestine points (gray dots)* 16, 17, 18, 19.

5. BIORHYTHM AND ENERGY FLUCTUATION

T HE CONCEPT OF BIORHYTHM, of an internal "biological clock" that regulates the organism's functioning in relation to both solar and lunar time measurement, is now an accepted part of Western physiology, particularly since problems caused by the disruption of this natural rhythm through jet travel over long distances—known as jet fatigue—have become a matter of concern.

Jet travel is new, but the ancient Chinese included the concept of biorhythm in their medical knowledge and used it in treatment. They distinguished not only the commonly recognized twenty-four-hour biorhythm but also biorhythms covering longer periods, eventually elaborating a biorhythmic pattern of wavelike curves of varying durations in order to measure exactly the fluctuations of energy circulation in the body.

The primary and most easily applied biorhythm used in acupuncture is that of the general circulation of energy within a twenty-four-hour period, each of the twelve regular meridians having a two-hour period of maximum energy flow as well as a two-hour period of minimum activity. The following timetable of the two-hour peak period for each of the twelve meridians is computed in sun hours, which vary from clock hours to a greater or lesser extent depending on geographical latitude and time of year.

Liver: 1–3 hours
Lungs: 3–5 hours
Large intestine: 5–7 hours
Stomach: 7–9 hours
Spleen-pancreas: 9–11 hours
Heart: 11–13 hours
Small intestine: 13–15 hours
Bladder: 15–17 hours
Kidneys: 17–19 hours
Heart constrictor: 19–21 hours
Triple heater: 21–23 hours
Gall bladder: 23–1 hours

This simple table represents the result of long and patient study of the times at which disorders involving the various organs regularly exhibit their most acute symptoms. Thus it can often be used in diagnosis to help establish what meridian is involved in a particular disorder and can also be used to treat a condition at the most favorable time. It is general knowledge that the worst asthma attacks take place during the small hours—the period of maximum activity in the lung meridian, according to the table. Such cases are most responsive to treatment between the third and fifth hours of the solar day. It has also been found that in the case of liver ailments characterized by paroxysms of pain or other symptoms regularly appearing at a specific time, it is most effective—in fact essential—to treat the ailment at the time of greatest liver meridian activity, between the first and third hours. This has been substantiated through extensive clinical experience by the authors.

A general rule of thumb handed down by tradition is that when treating a patient in accordance with this biorhythm, the best time to treat an excess of energy is at or shortly before the time of greatest meridian activity, while the best time to treat depleted energy is following the peak.

Many acupuncturists rely simply on this twenty-four-hour biorhythm, using the following timetable, which is memorized.

| | TO DISPERSE | | TO TONIFY | |
MERIDIAN	POINT	TIME	POINT	TIME
liver	2	1–3 hours	8	3–5 hours
lungs	5	3–5 hours	9	5–7 hours
large intestine	2	5–7 hours	11	7–9 hours
stomach	45	7–9 hours	41	9–11 hours
spleen-pancreas	5	9–11 hours	2	11–13 hours
heart	7	11–13 hours	9	13–15 hours
small intestine	8	13–15 hours	3	15–17 hours
bladder	65	15–17 hours	67	17–19 hours
kidneys	1	17–19 hours	7	19–21 hours
heart constrictor	7	19–21 hours	9	21–23 hours
triple heater	10	21–23 hours	3	23–1 hours
gall bladder	38	23–1 hours	43	1–3 hours

The second biorhythm used in acupuncture is that of the "hourly open points." Energy circulates through the body not only in relation to the sun hours of the day but also in relation to the Chinese lunar calendar, reaching a specific point at a particular two-hour period of a particular day within a ten-day cycle (see Appendix B). Just as the moon affects tides, plants, and other natural phenomena, so does it affect the human body. The old Chinese calendar, based on the phases of the moon, is divided into ten-day cycles composed of one yin and one yang day for each of the five elements: wood-yang, wood-yin, fire-yang, fire-yin, earth-yang, earth-yin, metal-yang, metal-yin, water-yang, and water-yin.

Each day is divided into twelve two-hour periods, each of which is identified with one of the twelve animals of the Chinese zodiac, as follows:

0–2 hours, rat
2–4 hours, ox
4–6 hours, tiger
6–8 hours, hare
8–10 hours, dragon
10–12 hours, snake
12–14 hours, horse
14–16 hours, sheep
16–18 hours, monkey
18–20 hours, cock
20–22 hours, dog
22–24 hours, boar

Years are also counted in a cycle of twelve, each year being identified with one of the twelve animals of the zodiac. Because the rotation of the days in the ten-day cycle is unvarying, it is possible to calculate the element and yin-yang categories of any day of a given year if one knows the categories of the first day of that year. One can also calculate the category of the first day of the next year, and so on. Following are the zodiacal and five-element designations for the first day of each year in the current twelve-year cycle.

1972: rat, metal-yin
1973: ox, fire-yin
1974: tiger, water-yang
1975: hare, fire-yin
1976: dragon, water-yang
1977: snake, earth-yang
1978: horse, water-yin
1979: sheep, earth-yang
1980: monkey, water-yin
1981: cock, earth-yin
1982: dog, water-yin
1983: boar, earth-yin

Knowing the categories of a given day, one can find the

hourly open point or points for any two-hour period on that day by referring to the chart in Appendix B. These are called hourly open points because they are open to maximum therapeutic effect at that time, being in their period of maximum energy potential within the ten-day cycle of general energy circulation. The Chinese explain the term "open point" by likening the energy in the body to irrigation water flowing through a system of canals (the meridians) with locks (the points). The best way to ensure a smooth flow of water through the canals is to open each lock just as the crest of the moving water reaches it. Likewise, the flow of energy in the body can be best regulated by treating points when they reach the period of maximum energy potential and are therefore most open to effective response to acupuncture. The acupuncturist using this biorhythm can use the various points to greatest therapeutic effect.

PART II

PRACTICE

6. DIAGNOSIS

ILLNESS, ACCORDING TO Chinese medicine, is basically nothing but a disturbance in the balance of body energy. This disturbance can be caused by external factors like excessive cold, heat, or humidity, or to internal factors like undernourishment, excessive emotion, anger, or fear. To treat a complaint, therefore, the Chinese practitioner pays less attention than his Western counterpart to the organ or organs involved and to the parts of the body manifesting symptoms, because reestablishment of the general balance of body energy will result in the abatement and disappearance of the symptoms. The Chinese consider the system involved rather than the specific organ showing morbid symptoms, the complainer rather than the complaint.

Diagnosis consists of establishing the relative imbalance of energy—in recognizing which meridians are exhibiting an excess and which a depletion of energy, and in identifying this as yin or yang energy. There are several methods of doing this, most of which reinforce one another: reading the pulses, palpation of abdominal points, and judicious observation and interrogation of the patient are among the most common.

PULSE DIAGNOSIS

The Chinese have elaborated the reading of the pulses as a diagnostic procedure to a degree unknown in Western medicine.

According to Chinese medicine, each of the twelve bilateral meridians is reflected in the radial artery and can be felt as a pulse at the wrist. There are three pairs of pulses on each wrist, at the following positions: *tsun,* between the fold of the wrist and the styloid protuberance; *kuan,* at the level of the styloid protuberance; and *ch'ih,* beyond the styloid protuberance (figs. 22 and 29). At each location two pulses can be palpated, one superficial (yang) and one deep (yin; fig. 23). In addition, the left wrist is considered yang and the right wrist yin; therefore the pulses of both wrists are palpated simultaneously (fig. 28).

Listed below are the pulses, their locations, and the meridians and organs that they reflect.

LEFT WRIST (YANG)
   tsun superficial: small intestine
   tsun deep: heart
   kuan superficial: gall bladder
   kuan deep: liver
   ch'ih superficial: bladder
   ch'ih deep: kidneys

RIGHT WRIST (YIN)
   tsun superficial: large intestine
   tsun deep: lungs
   kuan superficial: stomach
   kuan deep: spleen-pancreas
   ch'ih superficial: triple heater
   ch'ih deep: heart constrictor

The relative differences among the pulses indicate the state of energy balance within the body; reading the pulses reveals excess or depletion of the energy in the regular meridians and is therefore a *sine qua non* of diagnosis. (*Jen-mô, tu-mô,* and the six extraordinary meridians, being outside the general energy-circulatory system, are not reflected in the pulses.)

Generally, a "strong" pulse is considered a sign of possible excess. But the deciding factor is not the quality of any single pulse but the differences in intensity and quality of the pulses at all three wrist segments. In the West, the pulse is considered only in terms of frequency and strength of beat, the position at the wrist being of no particular significance. But in Chinese medicine, location is the key factor, for it is this that directly indicates which organs are being reflected in the pulses, and the organs' energy condition.

Other considerations include both quantitative and qualitative factors. Quantity (strength and frequency of the pulsebeat) is evaluated according to what is normal for the individual and in terms of overall strength. Among the criteria for judging normality are whether the yin pulses are stronger or weaker than the yang and whether the yin or yang pulse at one location is different from the pulses at other locations.

Quality is judged according to a complex set of criteria. Eighteen different qualities of the pulses are listed in Appendix C, together with their diagnoses and the type of acupuncture treatment indicated (stimulation or dispersal of energy).

ABDOMINAL DIAGNOSIS

Abdominal palpation is the most widely used form of diagnostic palpation in Chinese medicine. A disturbance of the energy balance within an organ is reflected along the entire length of its meridian and causes certain points of the meridian to become especially sensitive to pressure. The degree of sensitivity varies according to the individual. It is most variable at the points on the extremities; therefore these points are unsatisfactory for diagnosis. On the other hand, it is easiest to detect abnormal sensitivity on the points on the trunk of the body, particularly those on the abdomen. Because of this, palpation of these points can be used to confirm or nullify diagnosis by the pulses.

Generally, if the energy flow in a meridian is in excess there will be some rigidity of the muscles around its abdominal point or points, and the patient's sensitivity to pressure here will often be increased to the point of excruciating pain. If the meridian point or points on the abdominal wall show abnormally low sensitivity (hyposensitivity), pressure on the tissue around the

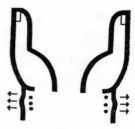

22. Pulse positions on the wrists. Tsun *is nearest the thumb,* kuan *is the middle position, and* ch'ih *is farthest from the thumb. There are two pulses at each position: a superficial, yang pulse and a deep, yin pulse. The dots indicate the five-element designations of the pulses at each position: (left) top, fire; middle, wood; bottom, water; (right) top, metal; middle, earth; bottom, fire.*

point or points will reveal a decrease in tone (atony). This is usually considered a sign of energy depletion.

Western medicine employs abdominal palpation in a manner superficially similar to that of Chinese medicine. But the Western physician is primarily interested in detecting pathology underlying the abdominal wall, while the Oriental practitioner is investigating the abdominal wall itself, focusing on meridian points. Therefore, while in Western practice the abdomen is examined with the patient's legs slightly flexed, in acupuncture diagnosis the legs are fully extended with no knee flexion, in order to maintain stretch on the abdominal wall.

The presence of a pain reaction at a meridian's abdominal points, most of which are bilateral, is not the only diagnostically significant element for the practitioner. The quality of pain indicates the yin or yang aspects of the energy-circulation imbalance. Pressure that elicits a clearly distressing pain reaction indicates an excess of yin energy. But if the opposite occurs, with the patient saying, for example, "It hurts—but it feels good," this is considered an indication of excessive yang energy. The rationale behind this is that yin causes expansion; pressure on the point increases expansion, so that the pain is increased. Yang causes contraction; pressure creates a form of expansion on the contracted part, thus providing a measure of relief.

In performing abdominal palpation, the practitioner passes his slightly warmed hand very lightly over the entire abdominal wall, seeking 1) areas of tightness or softness on the abdominal wall, 2) areas warmer or cooler than the surrounding surface, 3) areas of pain, and 4) the abdominal points of the meridians.

Though not all meridians cross the abdomen, all have associated diagnostic points on the front of the body trunk. Palpation of these will indicate areas of excess or depletion of yin and yang energy, and abdominal-point examination will define the problem area. This is then checked against the degree of tenderness evidenced on pressing the *gueki* point of the suspect meridian.

DIAGNOSIS BY OBSERVATION

The practitioner of Chinese medicine obtains many clues to the cause of a patient's distress by close observation of his general appearance, facial expressions, and voice. The lines on the face indicates character disposition and, with this, the tendency to particular organ dysfunctions. For example, vertical lines between the eyebrows are associated with irritability and quick anger, which involve the liver.

The general color of the face and other parts of the body also indicates organ involvement. Blackish coloring on the inside of the forearm, for instance, indicates kidney or bladder disturbance. (It should be borne in mind that the color changes mentioned in old Chinese and Japanese texts apply to Oriental pigmentation.)

The tone and quality of the patient's voice are also indicative of his general energy condition. Among the factors considered are whether the voice is strong or muffled, whether there is a sighing sound when speaking, and whether the main tone of the voice corresponds to any musical note. A strong, clear voice indicates abundant yang energy in a man, but in a woman this is considered to indicate a lack of yin energy, if there is an "aggressive" tone to the voice, so that the yang has become more evident.

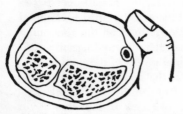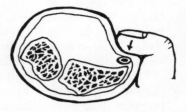

23. *Reading the yang and yin pulses. Light pressure is used to detect the yang pulses (left) and deep pressure to detect the yin pulses. According to the most ancient texts, the amount of pressure applied also varies according to the pulse position on the wrist.*

SYNDROMES: *CHENG*

Cheng (Japanese *sho*) corresponds to the English "syndrome" and means a group of symptoms that collectively shows what meridian or meridians to treat. Chinese medicine does not define pathological conditions as specific diseases, but the patient's *cheng* will correspond to a condition identified in Western medicine as a particular syndrome or disease.

The following list shows the areas and organs especially affected when the various meridians are involved. This knowledge helps in making and confirming diagnoses.

LUNG MERIDIAN: nose, throat, lungs

LARGE INTESTINE MERIDIAN: mouth, tongue, nose, face, ears, eyes, throat, esophagus, stomach

HEART CONSTRICTOR MERIDIAN: vascular system, thorax, stomach, heart, nerves

TRIPLE HEATER MERIDIAN: ears, eyes, shoulders, elbows, sides of chest

SMALL INTESTINE MERIDIAN: head, nape of neck, back, elbows

HEART MERIDIAN: heart, central nervous system

SPLEEN-PANCREAS MERIDIAN: intestines, stomach, liver, spleen, lungs

STOMACH MERIDIAN: viscera in general

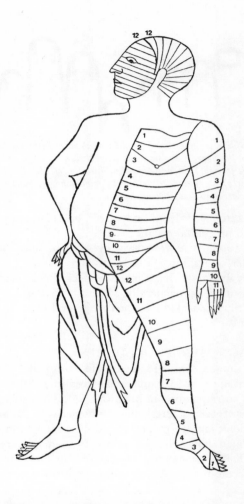

24. *Zones of Hirata: 1) bronchia, 2) lungs, 3) heart, 4) liver, 5) gall
bladder, 6) spleen-pancreas, 7) stomach, 8) kidneys, 9) large intestine, 10)
small intestine, 11) bladder, 12) genital organs.*

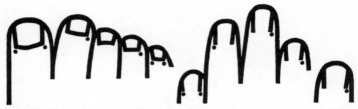

25. *The meridian terminal points used in Akabane's Test: big toe (left to right), spleen-pancreas, liver; second toe, stomach; fourth toe, gall bladder; fifth toe (left to right), kidneys, bladder; little finger (left to right), small intestine, heart; ring finger, triple heater; middle finger, heart constrictor; index finger, large intestine; thumb, lungs.*

LIVER MERIDIAN: sides of body, liver, gall bladder, pancreas, uterus, urogenital organs

GALL BLADDER MERIDIAN: ears, eyes, chest, sides, liver, gall bladder, knees, hips

BLADDER MERIDIAN: head, nape of neck, back, central nervous system, skin generally, viscera

KIDNEY MERIDIAN: kidneys, uterus, genital organs, bladder, throat

NEW DIAGNOSTIC PROCEDURES

ZONES OF HIRATA: In 1913 Kurakichi Hirata defined twelve zones covering the head, trunk, and extremities of the body and the organs corresponding to them (fig. 24). These zones are often the sites of eczemas, erethemas (reddened skin), or abnormal pigmentations, and the points located where these zones cross a meridian often show a marked sensitivity when that meridian is involved. This phenomenon can often resolve a diagnostic problem or indicate the specific treatment points in a given case.

AKABANE'S TEST: This test developed by Master Acupuncturist Kobe Akabane is not a classical acupuncture procedure but is based on meridian physiology. The terminal points of the bilateral meridians located at the corners of the fingernails and toenails (fig. 25) are stroked repeatedly, very lightly and rapidly, with the incandescent end of a burning incense stick until a pain response is elicited. A discrepancy in the number of strokes required on the right and left terminal points of the same bilateral meridian indicates an energy-circulation imbalance in that meridian.

A simpler procedure tests the relative sensitivity of the right and left terminal points of a bilateral meridian by applying equal pressure to both points with an implement having a blunt-pointed tip, such as the rounded end of a wooden match or toothpick, or the tip of a ballpoint pen.

7. THE NEEDLES AND THEIR USE

T HE PRIMARY, though not the only, technique of acupuncture treatment is the insertion of needles at meridian points. The earliest "needles" were fish bones, bamboo splinters, and pointed stones, which gave way to true needles made of such metals as iron and copper. At present, most needles are made of silver, gold, or stainless steel. Their shapes and sizes vary somewhat from country to country, and sometimes even from region to region, but are more or less standardized (figs. 30–32).

Some of the ancient Chinese masters of acupuncture attributed particular qualities to the metal or color of the needle: silver (white) was thought to aid in dispersing excess energy and gold (yellow) in stimulating or tonifying depleted energy. (Some modern experiments on the results of using gold and silver needles are described in Chapter 11.)

The acupuncturist considers type of metal, shape, diameter, and length of needle, as well as the treatment procedure to be used, in making his selection of needles. But regardless of the type of needle chosen, he is faced with one basic choice in treatment: to stimulate or to disperse the energy of the meridian. His procedures will vary, and with them his choice of needles, but his purpose will always be stimulation or dispersal—or sometimes both.

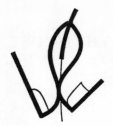

26. Placing the needle. The point of the needle is placed on the acupuncture point chosen for treatment, and the skin is pierced very lightly while the needle is held near its point.

Following are the general rules of energy control in acupuncture with the common type of needle.

TO STIMULATE:

1. Warm the needle (in former times the acupuncturist did this by holding the needle in his mouth for several minutes, but clearly this is no longer sanctioned).

2. Massage the point to be treated before inserting the needle.

3. Puncture superficially.

4. Introduce the needle slowly, in stages, and withdraw it slowly.

5. Puncture the points of the meridian in the same order as the direction of the flow of energy in the meridian.

6. Introduce the needle as the patient exhales and withdraw it as he inhales.

7. Keep the needle in place for three to ten minutes.

TO DISPERSE:

1. Use large needles.

2. Do not massage the point to be treated.

3. Insert the needle relatively deeply.

4. Introduce and withdraw the needle rapidly.

5. Puncture the meridian points in the opposite order of the direction of the flow of energy in the meridian.

6. Puncture as the patient inhales and withdraw as he exhales.

7. Leave the needle in place for only a few seconds.

8. Make the point bleed very slightly after withdrawing the needle (microbleeding).

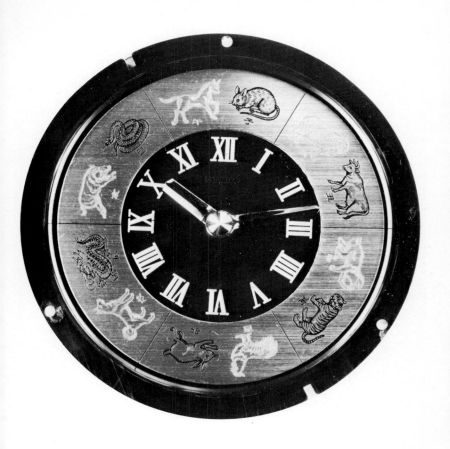

27. *The Chinese zodiacal clock. The signs of the Oriental animal zodiac indicate the twelve two-hour periods in a day. The white signs pertain to daytime hours, the black ones to nighttime hours.*

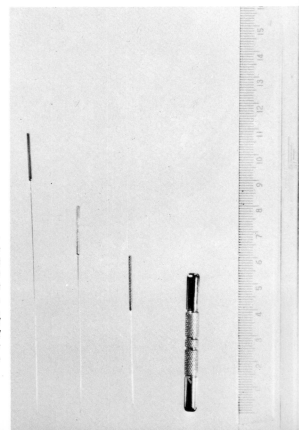

28. Taking the pulses. Both the right and left pulses are palpated at the same time. Numerous factors are considered and compared, such as strength and frequency of pulsebeat, quality of pulse (hesitant, tense, gliding, rough, and so on), and the relative yin-yang balance among the pulses.

30–32. Various types of acupuncture needles, with centimeter rules for size reference. From left to right: Japanese acupuncture needles and guide tube; Chinese acupuncture needles, including, left to right, intracutaneous needle, moxa needle, regular needle, and multiple-meridian needle (inserted so that it passes through two or more meridians); and Korean acupuncture needles.

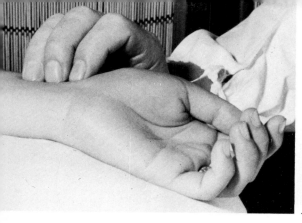

29. *Finger position in pulse-taking. The index finger is at* tsun, *the middle finger at* kuan, *and the ring finger at* ch'ih.

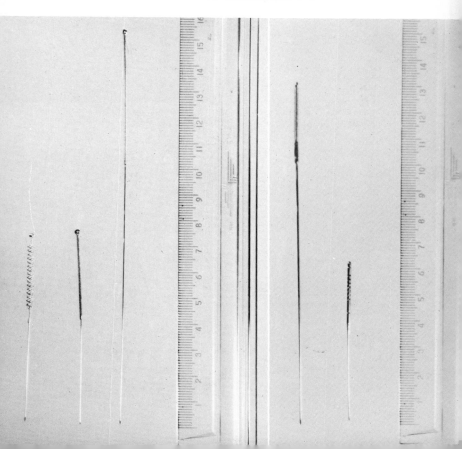

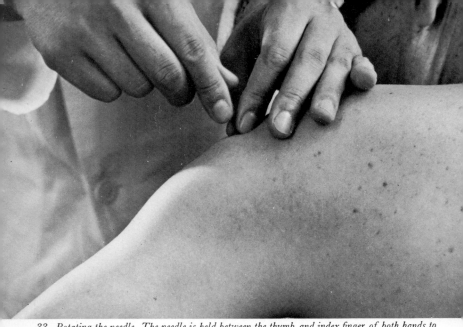

33. Rotating the needle. The needle is held between the thumb and index finger of both hands to execute this movement. Insertion of the needle is facilitated by rotating the needle head.

35. Using a small hammer. This is another Japanese ▷ technique, employed when no guide tube is used. The head of the needle is lightly tapped with the hammer to cause the point to penetrate the skin.

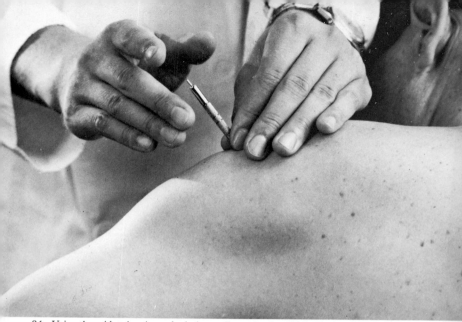

34. *Using the guide tube. A metal tube is usually used to introduce Japanese needles because they are so fine that they may bend otherwise. One end of the tube is placed on the point chosen for treatment, and the head of the needle is lightly tapped to cause the needle point to penetrate the skin.*

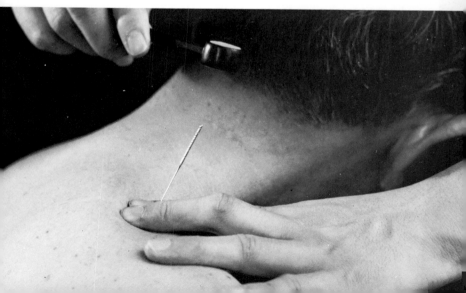

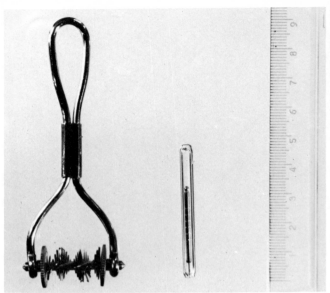

36. *Instruments for skin stimulation. The roller and the fine-pointed needle in a glass tube are most often used for cutaneous stimulation in the treatment of children.*

37. *Using the roller for skin stimulation.*

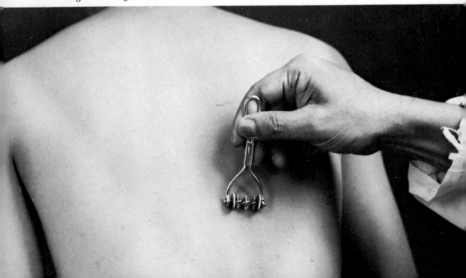

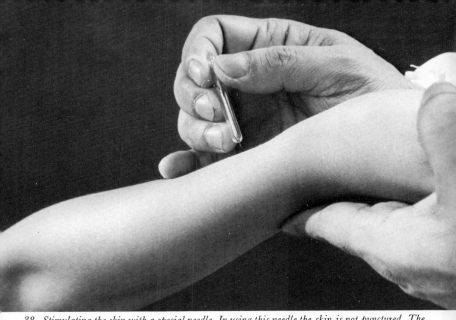

38. *Stimulating the skin with a special needle. In using this needle the skin is not punctured. The needle point is forced upward as the glass tube descends.*

39. *The Chinese "star needle." This is another stimulator, used with no penetration of the skin.*

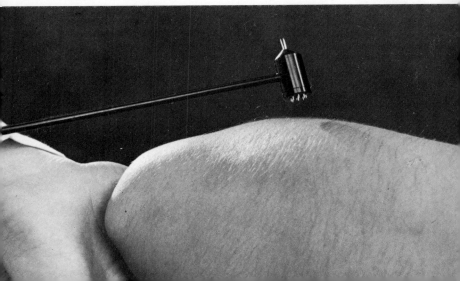

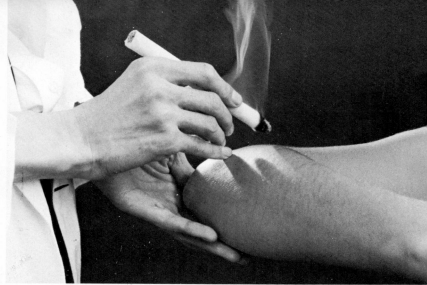

40. *A moxa stick. The burning moxa stick, or "cigarette," is held close to the treatment point until the patient's discomfort level is reached, when it is removed. The procedure is repeated many times in a treatment session. This method of moxibustion is favored by the Chinese.*

41. *A modification of the moxa stick.*

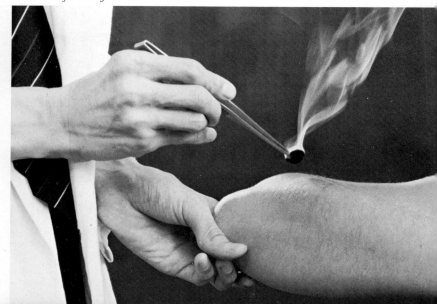

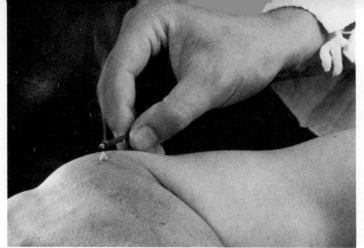

42. *Small moxa. A cone of moxa about the size of a rice grain is burned down to the skin. This is painful and produces a small blister. This method is very popular in Japan and is used extensively for home treatment.*

43. *Applying moxa via an acupuncture needle. There is no sensation of heat with this method, which is very effective in treating cases of energy depletion. It has been found to be superior to short-wave diathermy in relieving muscular pain and tightness.*

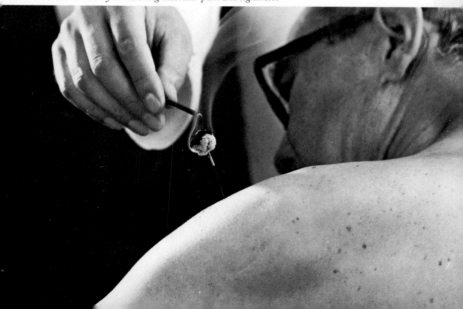

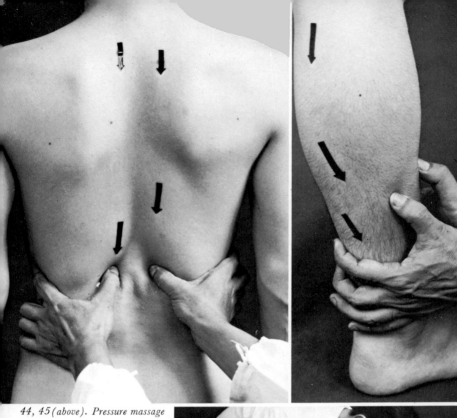

44, 45 (above). Pressure massage on back and leg. Arrows indicate the direction of the massage movements.

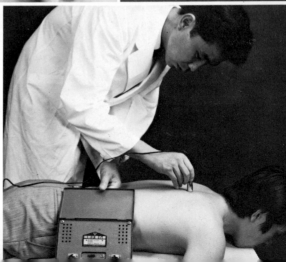

46. Nonscarring electric "moxa."

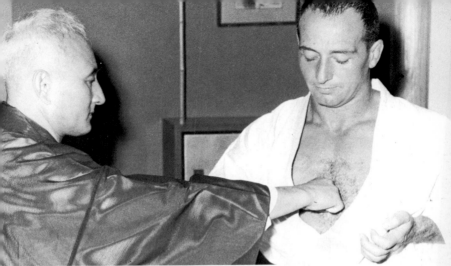

47. This and the following four photographs show the use of acupuncture points for self-defense. In this photograph the attacker's fist has been pushed aside, and a blow is being delivered to jen-mô *point 17* with the knuckle of the right index finger. This is most painful aud causes mild shock.

48. The attacker's thrust is thwarted by grasping his arm and applying pressure on heart *point 3* with the left thumb. This will cause the attacker to collapse.

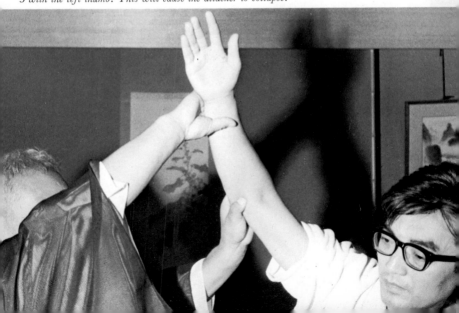

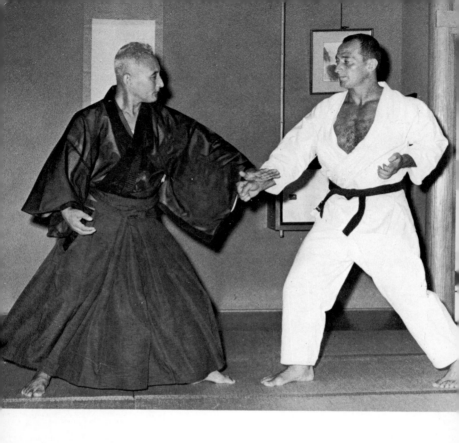

49–51. Three stages of one method of overpowering an opponent. First, an attack is stopped by chopping down on the assailant's fist (above). Pressure is then exerted on heart constrictor and triple heater points on the hand (opposite page, above). Pressure on these points is increased, using both hands, which renders the assailant helpless (opposite page, below).

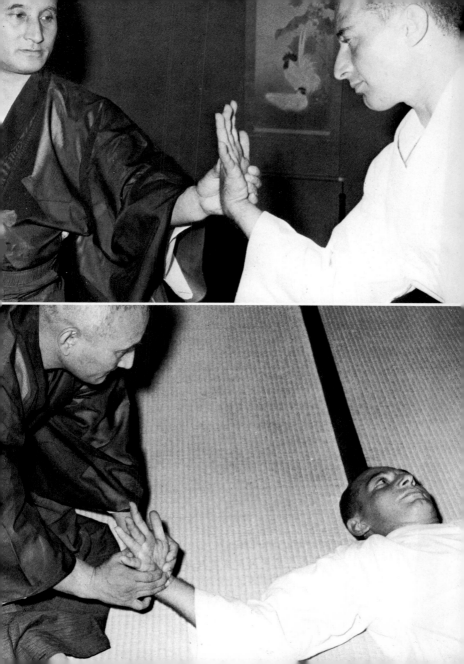

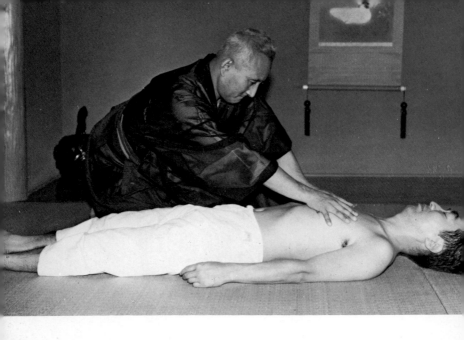

52–55. Katsu, *or resuscitation. One method of reviving an unconscious person using an acu-puncture point is shown here. First, stroke the victim lightly from chest to abdomen ten times (above). Then rest one leg on his back, rotating the knee slightly so that its point will not jut directly into the back, with the patella resting against a heart point on the back (opposite page, above). Finally, thrust repeatedly with the knee while pulling up and in on the right shoulder and pushing down on the left shoulder, with hands in the position shown (opposite page, below).*

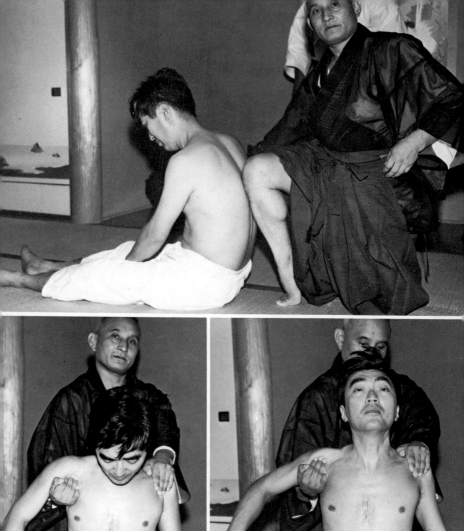
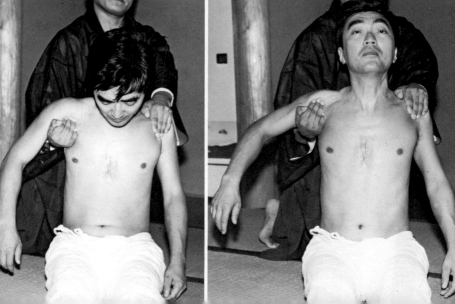

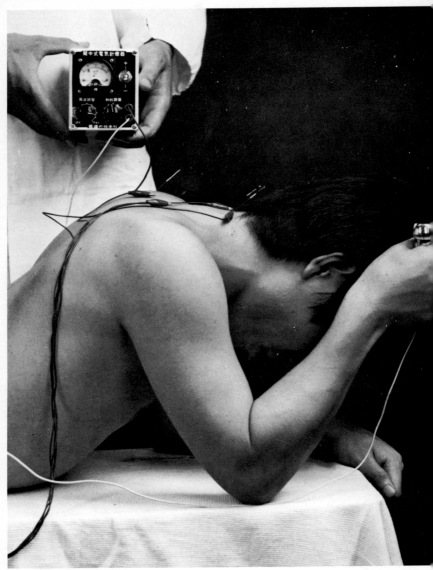

56. *Electrical acupuncture.*

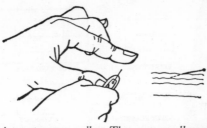

57. Inserting intracutaneous needles. These very small needles do not completely penetrate the skin but are lodged in the most superficial skin layer. They may be secured with adhesive tape and left in place for several days. The application technique requires the skin to be stretched with the fingers and then released against the needle, rather than the needle's being pushed into the skin.

Japanese needles are very delicate and are slid through a metal tube when inserted, to prevent their bending (fig. 34). The Chinese technique is to insert the needles without use of the guide tube (fig. 26).

No pain is felt in the insertion of even the largest acupuncture needles in the hands of a skilled practitioner. At most, a slight discomfort may occasionally be felt when the needle is inserted—but there should never be actual pain. Acupuncture students commonly practice extensively on themselves during their years of study in order to perfect their technique.

REACTIVE POINTS AND INTRACUTANEOUS NEEDLES

As its name suggests, the reactive point is the most sensitive point in a painful area. Puncturing at this point was without doubt the earliest acupuncture technique and can be remarkably effective in cases of pain, often producing immediate relief. The patient indicates the area of greatest pain, which is lightly probed until the most sensitive point is found. This is then punctured in dispersal. (This reactive point may or may not lie on a meridian.)

In Japan a variation of this technique uses tiny intracutaneous needles that can be left in place for a prolonged period. The patient is asked to indicate the most painful spot, which is marked. The intracutaneous needle is inserted there, penetrat-

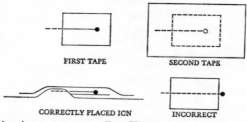

FIRST TAPE   SECOND TAPE

CORRECTLY PLACED ICN   INCORRECT

58. Securing intracutaneous needles. The needle head rests on a piece of adhesive tape; the entire needle is then covered with another piece of tape. There must be no pain or discomfort from these needles. If there is, it is the result of improper insertion, and the needle or needles must be removed at once.

ing only the first layer of skin, and held in place with adhesive tape (figs. 57 and 58). The patient then pinpoints the next most painful area, and the procedure is repeated; this continues as often as necessary. The needles remain until the next treatment.

The above method is used for localized pain. When dealing with pain over a large area, or when pain is accompanied by inflammation, swelling, or irritation of the skin, it is advisable to search for the most sensitive points on the periphery of the area, where intracutaneous needles are placed. Then the entire area is lightly and rapidly pricked without penetrating the skin.

MICROPUNCTURE

Whereas in premodern Western medicine bleeding took the barbaric form of draining the patient of considerable quantities of blood by the application of leeches, the Chinese directed a far gentler form of bleeding to specific points.

As the word "micropuncture" implies, the amount of blood drawn never exceeds a few drops—no more than would be withdrawn in an ordinary blood test. Frequently just one drop of blood removed at the appropriate acupuncture point will give immediate and startling results. For example, one drop withdrawn from the finger terminal point of the small intestine meridian will instantly relieve certain cases of pain from a stiff shoulder. Some types of headache, such as hangover headache, respond to the same procedure applied to the finger terminal of the large intestine meridian.

8. AUXILIARY TECHNIQUES:
MOXIBUSTION AND MASSAGE

MOXIBUSTION

THE BURNING OF MOXA, small cones of wormwood (*Artemisia vulgaris*), on the acupuncture points enjoys great popularity in Japan as a supplement to or even a substitute for needle therapy because moxa is very economical, can be self-administered, and is most effective in a cool, humid climate like Japan's. (This last is because in a cool, humid climate the energy circulates on a deeper level than in warmer, dryer regions. The heat of moxa has a penetrating effect, and if applied in the Oriental manner, raising a small blister, the stimulus is relatively long lasting.)

Moxa is a good deal simpler to apply than acupuncture needles. The cone is placed on the chosen point and ignited, usually by touching it with the burning end of an incense stick. There are three major types of moxa, each with a specialized application. Large moxas are about the size of a medium cherry, small moxas (fig. 42) about the size of a rice grain, and minute moxas about the size of the ball of a ballpoint pen.

Large moxas are usually used for stimulation of energy, though at times also for dispersal, and are removed when the patient indicates that the sensation of heat is uncomfortable. Their application can be repeated several times in one treatment session.

Small moxas are usually left to burn all the way down to the skin, which is very painful and produces a blister. These can be used for either stimulation or dispersal of energy and can also be applied repeatedly at one session.

Minute moxa, often applied in a series of a hundred or more, are used in special situations; they are also left to burn all the way down to the skin. If they have been correctly applied (that is, if the diagnosis and treatment chosen are correct), the burning will actually cause a pleasant sensation. When the patient complains of pain or discomfort from this kind of moxa application, the treatment has reached the point of maximum effect and the session is ended. The treatment may be repeated at another session, but this is seldom necessary.

In both China and Japan, moxa is often applied through a needle (fig. 43). The cone is placed on the end of a needle placed at an acupuncture point, and the heat of the moxa is conducted through the needle. This produces a very agreeable sensation. This technique is used most frequently for pain relief and is consistently effective in relief of muscular pain, as well as referred pain from internal organs.

MASSAGE

Oriental massage is a therapeutic procedure in its own right but is mentioned here because some massage manipulations are used in acupuncture as part of diagnostic palpation and are also frequently used very briefly before and after an acupuncture session. Oriental massage techniques appear to have aspects in common with Western methods, but the similarities are more in appearance than in purpose or effect.

Western massage is characterized by general centripetal friction directed at increasing blood circulation. Chinese and Japanese massage, on the other hand, are used in acupuncture to stimulate points or entire meridians by digital pressure, elbow pressure, stamping, scratching, and so on (figs. 44 and 45). Mobilization of the spinal column and of all joints is also part of this system of massage; these techniques are used in the treatment of children, the aged, and the extremely debilitated.

9. METHODS OF TREATMENT

THE VARIOUS diagnostic procedures considered indicate the degree and kind of energy imbalance in a given case: which meridians are carrying excess energy and which are in depletion, and whether this energy is yin or yang; the many relationships between yin and yang meridians on the whole; and the relationship between the energy circulation on the right and left sides of the body.

Once the kind and degree of energy imbalance have been analyzed, the acupuncturist will select one of several techniques to restore balance in accordance with the Chinese laws of physiology.

The first step is to reestablish the disturbed energy balance, then, should any symptom persist, to act directly on the point that is specific for the case in question. In examining some of the forms of treatment possible, we shall reverse this sequence, however, because of a traditional rule that in acute cases involving pain or fever this symptom must be treated first, then the general energy balance reestablished, should it still be necessary. This is because both pain and fever represent gross energy imbalances.

The imbalance of energy detected through diagnosis is a relative imbalance within a closed circuit; an excess of energy in one part or organ of the body reduces the energy in another part or organ by a corresponding amount, and vice versa. Pulse diagnosis indicates whether an excess is the cause of a depletion or whether a depletion has caused an excess—in other words, whether an excess or a depletion of energy is the primary cause of the imbalance. The ability to discern this is the mark of the true master of acupuncture.

To give an example: a pulse reading shows depletion at the *ch'ih* position on the left wrist and at the *tsun* position on the right wrist. Here a depletion of energy in water (bladder) and metal (large intestine) results in an excess in the opposing elements and their associated organs, wood (gall bladder) and fire (small intestine). In such a case, one stimulates the depleted meridians, which leads to a resultant depletion of energy in those meridians that are in excess.

An energy imbalance detected in diagnosis may be rectified by applying one or more of the following procedures: treatment by the law of the five elements, by the *lo* points, by the general yin-yang imbalance, by the "principle of opposites," and by the extraordinary meridians.

TREATMENT BY THE ELEMENT POINTS

Treatment according to the law of the five elements is based on the "mother-son" rule, as well as the affinities and antipathies between elements outlined in Chapter 3. The mother-son rule is the principle that an element is "son" of the one preceding it in the cycle of generation and "mother" of the one following it (fig. 3). This relationship naturally pertains also to the organs associated with the elements. Thus, the liver (wood) is mother of the heart (fire) and at the same time son of the kidneys (water). The heart constrictor and its coupled meridian, the triple heater, correspond to the element of fire. Following the mother-son rule, the heart constrictor is mother of the spleen-pancreas (earth) and son of the liver (wood). The triple heater is mother of the stomach (earth) and son of the gall bladder (wood).

The following examples show how this rule is applied in treatment on the element points of the meridians.

To disperse excess energy in the lung meridian we treat the water point of the lung meridian and the wood point of the kidney meridian. If the lung meridian is in a state of energy depletion, we stimulate the earth point of the lung meridian and the metal point of the liver meridian. The treatment is not yet complete, however, for we know that fire will destroy metal (fig. 4); that is, the heart can adversely affect the lungs. To prevent this, we treat the heart meridian in the opposite way to that in which we have treated the lung meridian. If we have dispersed the lung we stimulate the heart, and vice versa.

If a patient has an excess of energy in the spleen-pancreas meridian, there may be a corresponding depletion of energy in the liver. There is also an excess in the lung, though less than that in the spleen-pancreas, with an accompanying secondary depletion in the kidney and heart constrictor. Application of the law of the five elements will lead us to disperse the metal point of the spleen-pancreas and the water point of the lung and stimulate the water point of the liver and the metal point of the kidney.

After this procedure, the patient's pulses should be read once more, concentrating this time on the superficial, yang pulses. Should these indicate an imbalance with a pattern similar to the previous imbalance in the yin meridians, the same technique will be used, this time treating the same element points of the yang meridians that correspond to the yin meridians previously treated. Balance of energy should then be reestablished.

Should either an excess or a depletion of energy persist, we are faced with two options: 1) stimulate the origin point of the meridian if it is in depletion, or disperse the origin point if the meridian is in excess; 2) treat the *lo* points as described below.

TREATMENT BY THE *LO* POINTS

The *lo*, or passage, points join a deep, yin meridian and a superficial, yang meridian that are coupled at a pulse. There are twelve bilateral *lo* points: lung 7, large intestine 6, stomach 40, spleen-pancreas 4, heart 5, small intestine 7, bladder 58, kidney 4, heart constrictor 6, triple heater 5, gall bladder 37, and liver 5. The *jen-mô* and *tu-mô* meridians also have *lo* points, *jen-mô* 1 and *tu-mô* 1.

These points are utilized to balance two coupled meridians when one is in depletion and the other in excess. Theoretically, one can either disperse the *lo* point of a meridian in excess or stimulate that of a meridian in depletion, but clinical experience has shown the second course to be preferable, because stimulation is a safer procedure than dispersal. Stimulation of the appropriate meridian will result in dispersal of an excess in another meridian because of the law by which an excess in one meridian is offset by a corresponding depletion in a meridian of an opposing element.

In an example of this procedure, to balance the meridians of the stomach and spleen-pancreas, with the former in excess and the latter in depletion, we stimulate the *lo* point of the spleen-pancreas. By taking the pulses, we can determine when the two are balanced. If after a few moments the pulses are not yet in balance, we stimulate the origin point of the spleen-pancreas, which should bring the pulses into balance.

TREATMENT OF YIN-YANG IMBALANCE

When a pulse reading indicates that all the yin or all the yang meridians are in either excess or depletion, it is necessary to act on the yin and yang meridians as groups. Several procedures are available: 1) stimulate the *lo* points of all the yang meridians if these are in depletion, or the *lo* points of all the yin meridians should these be in depletion; 2) stimulate the *lo* point of *jen-mô* to treat a depletion in the yin meridians, or the *lo* point of *tu-mô* for the same condition in the yang meridians; 3) stimulate the master points of the four yin extraordinary meridians (*jen-mô* is here considered an extraordinary meridian) for a deficiency of energy in the yin regular meridians, or the master points of the four yang extraordinary meridians (including *tu-mô*) to treat a depletion in the yang regular meridians.

Should the pulses remain unbalanced after this treatment, a number of other procedures can be used. Pricking the origin points is usually the most effective alternate treatment.

It must be remembered that fever in a patient, no matter what its cause, should be treated before trying to rectify a general yin-yang imbalance, because fever represents in itself a serious general yin-yang imbalance that will persist unless the fever is reduced. The same is true of extreme pain. Acupuncturists consider the following points to be specific for fevers: under the third dorsal vertebra for fever of thoracic origin, under the fourth dorsal vertebra for fever of epigastric origin, under the fifth dorsal vertebra for fever caused by the liver, under the sixth dorsal vertebra for fever caused by the spleen-pancreas, and under the seventh dorsal vertebra for fever of renal origin. When a fever cannot be attributed to any of the above causes, one or more of the following points should be pricked in dispersal: gall bladder 20, gall bladder 34, bladder 11, bladder 12, large intestine 4, and *tu-mô* 19.

TREATMENT BY "PRINCIPLE OF OPPOSITES"

Disorders manifesting symptoms on the posterior aspect of the body are often most effectively treated on the anterior aspect of the body, and vice versa. Lumbago back pain, for example, can be treated by stimulating the sensitive points of the thorax and abdomen. In the case of stomach disturbance, one can treat the *tu-mô* or *iu* points of the stomach, which are on the back.

In accordance with this "principle of opposites," one should also treat complaints of the upper body by points on the lower body, and vice versa. Complaints affecting the trunk of the body can be treated on either the limbs or the trunk, as well as by stimulation of points on the meridian crossing the area that exhibits symptoms.

The "great *piqure,*" or great puncture, is advised in treating pain and unilateral symptoms (symptoms appearing on only one side of the body). After locating the most sensitive point on the meridian that crosses the involved area, the corresponding point on the unaffected side of the body is treated.

TREATMENT BY EXTRAORDINARY MERIDIANS
When there is an excess of energy, as in febrile diseases and cases involving pain, one or more of the extraordinary meridians become activated; a balance of energy can then be attained only by acting on these meridians. Pressure on several points of each extraordinary meridian, especially the one that coincides with the pain trajectory, will establish which meridian is involved, as this one will manifest several painful points.

Two treatment procedures are possible. One is to place needles on two points of the meridian, a gold needle on that nearest the meridian's origin and a silver needle on the one closest to its terminus (the use of gold and silver needles is discussed in Chapter 11). For example, if the meridian involved is *yang-oe,* one may puncture with a gold needle bladder 63 or gall bladder 35, these two being at the starting point of the meridian, and puncture with a silver needle large intestine 14 or gall bladder 21, which are closer to the end of the meridian. The other procedure is to puncture the meridian's master point with gold and the master point of its coupled meridian with silver. In the case of *yang-oe,* the gold needle would be placed on the master point of *yang-oe,* triple heater 15, and the silver needle on gall bladder 41, the master point of *tae-mo.*

Treatment on the extraordinary meridians is usually instituted only when treatment of the regular meridians is not effective, which is in itself an indication of involvement of the extraordinary meridians.

PEDIATRICS
Acupuncture applied to children differs in several respects from that used with adults. For one thing, light stimulation of the

meridians by massage or scratching, with no insertion of needles, usually suffices because children respond much more quickly than adults. Confronted also with the difficulty of establishing a diagnosis from a child's pulses, it is necessary to apply generalized treatment, often by gently scratching the length of a meridian for four or five minutes. This technique is used especially along the meridians on the trunk.

This very simple form of treatment gives remarkable results with nervousness, enuresis (incontinence of urine), insomnia, digestive or appetite upsets, and anorexia (loss of appetite). Quite often an asthma crisis can be prevented by lightly scratching the arms along the meridians of the large intestine and/or the lungs, or the legs along the kidney meridian, using a blunt-pointed instrument.

PRECAUTIONARY MEASURES

Several acupuncture points can be dangerous if used injudiciously. They are used only by a master acupuncturist and then only with extreme caution and only in conjunction with action on certain other points that have a controlling effect on the dangerous ones.

The general energy condition of a patient should always be taken into consideration when determining any treatment procedure, and utmost care should be taken not to lower this further. For this reason, although dispersal of energy is simpler and acts more rapidly than stimulation, it should be applied only with great caution. Stimulation properly applied will disperse excess energy in another meridian, whereas dispersal does not lead to as much counterbalancing stimulation and therefore tends to result in a general lowering of the patient's energy level. When the stomach is in excess, for example, stimulation properly applied to the lung or large intestine meridian will disperse the stomach's excess.

In addition to these general precautions, several procedures are observed to prevent untoward happenings during treatment.

1. Disinfect needles with alcohol.
2. Examine needle points carefully for breakage.
3. Have the patient lie down, as the possibility of adverse reaction to the needles is decreased.
4. Do not administer micropuncture or leave needles in place in the following cases: heart disease, anemia, hemorrhage, following childbirth or mental shock, or when the patient is hypersensitive, intoxicated, angry, very hungry, aged, or a young child.
5. Inquire how the patient is feeling during treatment, and watch for cold sweats, changes of color, and nausea.
6. Micropuncture must not cause a strong pain response or much bleeding. Massage applied beforehand will prevent pain.
7. Do not have needles in other parts of the body when working on the head.
8. Do not move needles on other parts of the body while working on the fingers.

Should the patient faint despite all precautionary measures, he can be revived by pressing the central nasolabial groove just under the nostrils, by puncturing spleen-pancreas 1, or by applying *katsu* resuscitation techniques (figs. 52–55).

10. THE EFFICACY OF ACUPUNCTURE

THE DEGREE of chronicity of a pathological condition affects both the duration and the efficacy of acupuncture treatment. Generally speaking, the longer a condition has been established before commencement of acupuncture therapy, the longer the treatment required and the more attenuated or problematical its efficacy. Nevertheless, spectacular results can be achieved even in chronic cases, as the three case histories on page 127 demonstrate. Generally speaking, the greater the organic involvement, the longer is treatment necessary. In patients responsive to acupuncture, from one to six visits are required. In slow cases, as many as twenty visits may be necessary. Paralysis is the most difficult of all forms of energy depletion to rectify and responds most slowly, though even this varies considerably with the individual.

In cases involving pain, daily treatment is required until this symptom subsides. In chronic cases without pain, at least two visits a week are required. In Japan, as mentioned earlier, the patient will often used self-administered moxa between or even in lieu of acupuncture sessions after the first treatment.

After the initial treatment there is often an aggravation of the symptoms, followed by a distinct improvement. In other cases there is an immediate improvement after the first treatment, but the following day the symptoms become more marked. In the latter case, the points treated should be modified.

Acupuncture has three major effects: 1) *sedation,* without unpleasant side effects like those accompanying drug sedation; 2) *relaxation,* produced by control of the hypotonicity or hyperactivity of organs; and 3) *functional modifications,* which include the regulation of excessive bleeding (hemostasis), of weight (obesity and underweight), of mental depression or excitation, of a general susceptibility to disease, and of insomnia, diarrhea, colds, constipation, menstrual disorders (excessive bleeding, lack of bleeding, and difficult or painful menses), impotence, premature ejaculation, and other problems of sexual functioning.

A number of disorders are listed below according to their degree of responsiveness to acupuncture. In group A acupuncture is very effective, in group B effective, in group C inconsistent, and in group D provides only symptomatic relief.

A. Headaches, head congestion, contusions, cramps (muscular, intestinal, and uterine), muscular pain, depression, referred pain, fatigue, hemorrhoids, neuralgia, nervous disorders in children, and the first phases of such inflammatory disorders as abscesses, appendicitis, and pneumonia.

B. Diarrhea, dysmenorrhea (painful or difficult menses), eczema, gastric hyperacidity, hypotension, kidney or gall bladder dysfunction, nervous disorders, palpitations, facial paralysis, prolapsed anus, rheumatism, shingles, and functional problems in the autonomic nervous system, especially following surgery.

C. Angina pectoris, arthritis, asthma, beri-beri, diabetes, renal hypertension, insomnia, kidney disease, trigeminal neuralgia, paralysis, vomiting, and stomach ulcers.

D. Tuberculosis, cancer, hemiplegia, infantile paralysis, and Parkinson's disease.

Acupuncture is ineffective following therapy involving X-rays, morphine, cortisone, or tranquilizers, because these affect the body in such a way as to modify drastically the normal rhythm of energy circulation. Electrical testing has revealed that in such cases the usual wavelike pattern of energy circulation in the meridians flattens out.

Following are three case histories that demonstrate the effectiveness of acupuncture in the treatment of chronic ailments.

Case A: businesswoman, 38. For three years she had had chronic pain in her left ankle treated at three different hospitals as rheumatic arthritis or gout, but with no improvement. Careful observation by an acupuncturist revealed that the disorder originated in the kidney meridian, not the ankle. Three acupuncture treatments cleared up the problem permanently.

Case B: man, 44. He suffered from chronic hepatitis, accompanied by urticaria (nettle rash) that appeared every night for about four years. Hospital treatment cured the hepatitis, but the nightly urticaria persisted. Reading the pulses in the Chinese manner revealed a deficiency in the liver meridian, which was treated by acupuncture. After seven treatments the urticaria disappeared permanently.

Case C: farmer, 66. For thirteen months he had suffered from a nightly fever of unknown origin that reached a peak of 100 to 102 degrees Fahrenheit (38 to 39 degrees centigrade) around midnight. Several physicians examined him but could not determine the fever's cause, and no Western medical treatment, including cortisone, was effective. The pulses revealed a deficiency in the liver meridian, but regular acupuncture treatment was ineffective. Then the same treatment was applied in accordance with the twenty-four-hour timetable of maximum meridian activity, upon which the fever disappeared permanently.

59. An old woodcut indicating acupuncture points for use in veterinary medicine.

11. INDICATIONS FOR THE FUTURE: NEW RESEARCH IN ACUPUNCTURE

THAT ACUPUNCTURE is neither superstition nor a purely psychosomatic therapy is attested by the fact that it has been widely and successfully used with domestic animals, such as horses, cattle, and camels. The most marked difference between veterinary and human acupuncture is that the former makes no use of meridians as such but only of specific points, which are acted on by bleeding, cauterization, and insertion of needles (fig. 59). As there is obviously no psychosomatic or placebo effect with animals, we can safely assert that acupuncture does work. Just how it works is a much more difficult question to answer.

Some indication that physiological laws as yet imperfectly understood are at work in acupuncture can be seen from the press reports from the People's Republic of China, Japan, and many other countries. Open-chest surgery has been successfully performed with acupuncture providing the only anesthetic. Through acupuncture, impaired hearing and color blindness have been rectified, and appendicitis has been relieved without surgery.

Acupuncture is presently practiced to greatest effect in the People's Republic of China, for in addition to the advantage afforded by the knowledge accumulated over thousands of years, the present government has taken the realistic attitude that if acupuncture works it should be studied and applied even at the risk of shattering established scientific theories. Acupuncture is now officially recognized as a valid therapy and is practiced in conjunction with Western medical techniques.

The Soviet Union also has well-established research and clinical programs in acupuncture, while scores of physicians in other countries are pursuing independent research in this field (see Appendix E).

A few of the recent experiments and findings in acupuncture research are outlined below to indicate the potential for its further development and wider application in the future. Here we discuss only Japanese research, not because it is necessarily superior to that in other nations but because the authors can report from first-hand experience and observation.

One of the modern advances in acupuncture has been the development of electrical instruments to detect the acupuncture points and objectively measure their properties (fig. 56). There are a number of such instruments, developed by several researchers in various countries: Niboyet in France, Lanza in Italy, Nakatani and Manaka in Japan, and others.

When measuring the impedance (resistance to passage of an electric current) of the terminal points of meridians with an electrical detector, differences are registered between the terminal points of the left and right branches of the same meridian, as well as between the terminal points of different meridians on the same side of the body. Through this phenomenon the difference between the left and right branches of a meridian, which is very difficult to establish through reading the pulses, is clarified. All other considerations aside, this alone renders the systematic use of electrical testing of the greatest importance.

Much research in this area is under way in both Europe and Asia, and it is hoped that an apparatus will soon be developed that will give consistent readings, allowing truly objective diagnoses of energy imbalance and thus assuring a higher percentage of successful treatments. In using this procedure, however, it must be kept in mind that the hourly general circulation of energy will disturb the reading for the terminal points of a meridian that is in its period of maximum energy activity at the time of the test. Nevertheless, on the basis of present knowledge it seems safe to say that electrical testing of the impedance of the terminal points can replace pulse examination in cases where the pulses are difficult to differentiate.

In experiments made to balance the impedance of the terminal points, a phenomenon has occurred that appears to indicate that the metal of which an acupuncture needle is made does affect the reaction elicited. The terminal points were tested electrically, and the meridian revealing the greatest difference in the impedance of the terminal points on the left and right branches was singled out. On the branch showing the greater impedance on the detector, a gold and a silver needle were placed a few centimeters apart, near the terminal point. When the gold needle was nearer the terminal point, the impedance registered by the two branches became balanced. But when the silver needle was nearer the terminal point, the difference in impedance was unaffected. Without drawing any definite conclusions regarding this phenomenon, it does seem to indicate that the results of acupuncture differ according to the metal of the needles and in relation to the direction of energy circulation in the meridian.

The same balancing effect has been obtained by placing two tiny metal contacts about one square millimeter in size, one of iron and one of copper, near a selected point. In cases of pain on a limb or in the abdomen, placement of the two metal contacts has been sufficient to obliterate it. Yet when the positions of the two contacts are reversed vis-à-vis the same pain area, the pain returns. This phenomenon is still under investigation.

Several experimental projects focus on pain relief and its relation to the general yin-yang energy balance. The pain-obliteration effect of the two-metal-contact experiment has led to further experiments in this area. One of these, the ion-flow experiment, deals with deep pain, such as chest or lumbago pain. A silver needle is placed on a yin meridian on the arm and another on a yin meridian on the leg. The needles are joined by a wire incorporating a germanium insert (germanium allows current to flow in one direction only). When the body-energy current is allowed to flow from arm to leg, there is no effect on the pain; but when the connecting wire is reversed so that the current flows from leg to arm, the deep pain subsides. This effect is markedly enhanced when magnets are placed in contact with the patient. This and other experiments suggest that whereas Western medicine deals with body chemistry, the principles at work in acupuncture have to do with body physics.

A crucial question in any consideration of acupuncture is whether energy, in the sense of the Chinese *ch'i*, exists. The authors think that experiments like those described above demonstrate that it does, though much more work needs to be done in this area. Corollary question are: if energy exists, does it really flow, and does it do so as traditionally specified?

It has been found that the activity of the meridians as registered on electrical equipment does indeed fluctuate in two-hour periods more or less as described in the ancient texts. This fact has been successfully used in the treatment of patients whose diagnosis and treatment according to both Western and Chinese medicine were unsatisfactory, like the farmer whose case was described in Chapter 10. In all such cases, it has been found that one or two meridians grossly deviated from the norm; when these were treated by acupuncture in accordance with the twenty-four-hour biorhythm of peak meridian activity, the conditions were rectified.

The experiments outlined above indicate that, old as it is as a practical therapy, the true potential of the science of acupuncture is only beginning to be realized. If investigated and applied in a spirit of truly dispassionate scientific inquiry, the prospects of acupuncture as a therapeutic system are promising indeed.

APPENDICES

APPENDIX A

Command Points of the Bilateral Meridians

This table lists the ten major points for control of the energy flow in each of the twelve bilateral meridians. Its application in treatment is governed by specific laws, which are discussed in the text. Following are the abbreviations used for the various meridians: lung—L, large intestine—LI, stomach—S, spleen-pancreas—SP, heart—H, small intestine—SI, bladder—B, kidney—K, liver—Li, gall bladder—GB, triple heater—TH, heart constrictor—HC, *jen-mô*—JM, *tu-mô*—TM.

	WOOD	FIRE	EARTH	METAL
LUNG	L 11	L 10	L 9	L 8
LARGE INTESTINE	LI 3	LI 5	LI 11	LI 1
STOMACH	S 43	S 41	S 36	S 45
SPLEEN-PANCREAS	SP 1	SP 2	SP 3	SP 5
HEART	H 9	H 8	H 7	H 4
SMALL INTESTINE	SI 3	SI 5	SI 8	SI 1
BLADDER	B 65	B 60	B 54	B 67
KIDNEY	K 1	K 2	K 6	K 7
LIVER	Li 1	Li 2	Li 3	Li 4
GALL BLADDER	GB 41	GB 38	GB 34	GB 44
TRIPLE HEATER	TH 3	TH 6	TH 10	TH 1
HEART CONSTRICTOR	HC 9	HC 8	HC 7	HC 5

WATER	ORIGIN	LO	GUEKI	ALARM	IU
L 5	L 9	L 7	L 6	L 1	B 13
LI 2	LI 4	LI 6	LI 7	S 25	B 25
S 44	S 42	S 40	S 34	JM 12	B 21
SP 9	SP 3	SP 4	SP 8	Li 13	B 20
H 3	H 7	H 5	H 6	JM 14	B 15
SI 2	SI 4	SI 7	SI 6	JM 4	B 27
B 66	B 64	B 58	B 63	JM 3	B 28
K 10	K 3	K 4	K 5	GB 25	B 23
Li 8	Li 3	Li 5	Li 6	Li 14	B 18
GB 43	GB 40	GB 37	GB 36	GB 24	B 19
TH 2	TH 4	TH 5	TH 7	B 5	B 22
HC 3	HC 7	HC 6	HC 4	unknown	B 14

APPENDIX B

Hourly Open Points

It will be noticed that two points are shown in many of the hour-day squares in the chart below. These are the principle and secondary points. It is beyond the scope of this book to give all the laws that apply to determining which is the principle point; in practice both points can be used. In time periods with only one point shown, no decision is required in point selection. All the hourly points of a given time period are thought to be particularly active at that time, regardless of the diagnosis of the case under consideration.

	WATER (Yin) 癸		WATER (Yang) 壬		METAL (Yin) 辛		METAL (Yang) 庚		EARTH (Yin) 己	
GALL BLADDER		○TH	▲LI			■S	□SI			●GB
LIVER	○K			□HC	■SP			□H		●Li
LUNG	□Li	□L	●B	○B		■TH	▲S			■SI
LARGE INTESTINE	□Li		■L	□LI	○L	▲L		○HC		■H
STOMACH	■LI	○S	●GB	□GB	■S	○S	●LI	○LI		●TH
SPLEEN-PANCREAS	■HC		■S	○SP	□K	●K	●S	○SP	○SP	▲SP
HEART	○S		▲TH	△B △TH ▲SI	●SP	■H	■B	□B	●SP	■H
SMALL INTESTINE	●H	■SI	▲H		●HC	■Li ■L	▲H	■SI	□L	●L
BLADDER	□LI		●S		○SI		□TH	▲LI △GB	▲SI	▲B
KIDNEY	○B	▲K	●SP			○H	▲LI		▲HC	■SP ■K
HEART CONSTRICTOR	▲B			■LI	□S			●SI		○GB
TRIPLE HEATER		▲K	■L			□SP	●H			○Li

KEY TO SYMBOLS

- ● = fire
- ■ = earth
- ○ = metal
- □ = water
- ▲ = wood
- △ = origin point

EARTH (Yang) 戊		FIRE (Yin) 丁		FIRE (Yang) 丙		WOOD (Yin) 乙		WOOD (Yang) 甲		
○ TH		△ SI	▲ LI	■ S			□ SI	● GB		子 0–2 RAT
	○ K	□ HC		■ LI	■ SP	□ H			● Li	丑 2–4 OX
□ Li	□ L	○ B	● B	■ TH		△ GB	▲ S	■ SI		寅 4–6 TIGER
	□ Li	■ L	□ LI	▲ L	○ L	○ HC		■ HC	■ K ■ H	卯 6–8 HARE
■ LI	○ S	□ GB	■ GB	■ LI	○ S	○ LI	● LI	■ TH		辰 8–10 DRAGON
	■ HC	● S	○ SP	● K	□ K	● S	○ SP	▲ SP	○ SP	巳 10–12 SNAKE
	○ S	▲ SI	▲ TH	● SP	■ H	□ B	■ B	● SP	■ H	午 12–14 HORSE
▲ H	■ SI		▲ H	■ Li	● HC	▲ H	■ SI	● L	□ L	未 14–16 SHEEP
	□ LI	● S			○ SI	▲ GB	□ TH	▲ SI	▲ B	申 16–18 MONKEY
○ B	▲ K		● SP	○ H			▲ Li	■ K	▲ HC	酉 18–20 COCK
	△ B ▲ B	■ LI			□ S	● SI			○ GB	戌 20–22 DOG
▲ K			■ H ■ L	□ K				● H	○ LI	亥 22–24 BOAR

APPENDIX C

Pulse Qualities

	QUALITIES	DIAGNOSIS	ACTION
	1 DELUGE swollen, powerful, superficial	fever, superficial complaint—fullness of yang	disperse
	2 ONION STALK swollen, soft	hemorrhage, fatigue	stimulate
	3 FLOATING superficial, floating	fever, superficial complaint	stimulate
	4 EMPTY superficial, slow, soft	decrease of yin	stimulate
	5 SOFT small, hard to find	decrease of yin	stimulate
	6 FULL swollen, powerful, large	fullness of HC and TH	disperse
	7 CHOKED strong, deep	constipation—fullness of yin	disperse
	8 PRISON strong, deep, wide	serious symptom: edema, nephritis, heart condition	disperse
	9 ROPE stretched	liver and bile complaints, epigastric pain, headaches—fullness	disperse

QUALITIES	DIAGNOSIS	ACTION
10 WEAK deep, soft	decrease of energy, malnutrition, palsy	disperse
11 VERY DEEP pulse on the bone	temporary change of fullness	disperse
12 RAPID more than five beats to one respiration	fever	disperse
13 STRETCHED irregular, unbalanced	fever, abscess	disperse
14 SLIDING	lack of energy	disperse
15 PRESSING frequent skipping	serious symptom: fullness of yang and lack of yin	stimulate yin
16 LENGTHENED fourth pulse can be felt beyond *ch'ih*	fullness of yin, pregnancy	stimulate
17 SLOW	cold, strong pain, general weakness	stimulate
18 NORMAL		

APPENDIX D
Organ-Element Concordances

	WOOD	FIRE	EARTH	METAL	WATER
ORGANS*	liver, gall bladder	heart, small intestine	spleen-pancreas, stomach	lungs, large intestine	kidneys, bladder
PLANET	Jupiter	Mars	Saturn	Venus	Mercury
DIRECTION	east	south	center	west	north
CLIMATE	windy	warm	humid	dry	cold
MAXIMUM ACTIVITY	spring	summer	late summer	fall	winter
COLOR	green	red	yellow	white	black
TASTE	sour	bitter	sweet	acrid	salty
ODOR	rancid	burned	perfumed	smoked	putrid
INCLINATION	tears	sweat	salivation	sobs	expectoration
EXPRESSIVE REACTION	noisiness	laughter	song	fearfulness	groaning
HARMFUL SENTIMENTS	euphoria	dissatisfaction	obsession	anxiety	fear
FOODS	millet, mutton	wheat, chicken	rye, beef	rice, horse	beans, pork
BODY TISSUE	muscle, tendons	blood vessels	flesh**	skin, hair	bone
SENSOR CONTROLLED	eyes	tongue	mouth	nose	ears

* The heart constrictor and triple heater are not included because they are not organ structures.

** Flesh includes such body tissues as tendons, fasciae, ligaments, and fat.

APPENDIX E

Presidents of Acupuncture Associations

(as listed in the *Nouvelle revue internationale
d'acupuncture*, April–June, 1971)

ARGENTINA: Dr. Sussman, Tucuman 1-762, Buenos Aires; president of the Argentine Acupuncture Association

AUSTRIA: Dr. Bischko, Tivoligasse 65, Vienna 12; president of the Austrian Acupuncture Association

BELGIUM: Dr. Baesens, 50 rue Stanley, Brussels

BRAZIL: Dr. Spaeth, Av. Copacabana 1-138, Rio de Janeiro

CANADA: Dr. Saita, 24 Clyde Medical Centre, 659 Clyde Ave., Park Royal, West Vancouver, B.C.

CZECHOSLOVAKIA: Dr. Richard Umlauf, Volenska Nemdenica, 5 N.P. Ruzemberok, Matrozovova 10; president of the Acupuncture Association
Dr. Georges Soukup, Navysinach 22, Prague; overseas secretary

FRANCE: Dr. Mommier, 23 rue Clapeyron, Paris 8; president of the International Acupuncture Association

GREECE: Dr. Trangas, 25 rue Julianou, Athens; president of the Hellenic Acupuncture Association

HONG KONG: Dr. Leung Kok Yuen, 322 King's Road, North Point; president of the Chinese Acupuncture Association

INDIA: Dr. Abdul Jalil, Institute of History of Medicine and Medical Research, Hamdard Building, Asaf Ali Road, New Delhi

INDONESIA: Dr. C. Hembing, Widjaja Kesuma, The Acupuncture Therapy Clinic, Djalan Taruma 48, Medan, Sumatra

ISRAEL: Dr. Louis Grunwald, 22 rue Balfour, Bat Yam; president of the Israel Acupuncture Association

ITALY: Dr. Uldérico Lanza, Torre Pellice, Via XX Settembre, Turin; president of the Italian Acupuncture Association

JAPAN: Dr. Sodo Okabe, 1-50, 3-chome, Kamiuma-machi, Setagaya-ku, Tokyo; president of the Japanese Acupuncture and Moxibustion Association
Dr. Haruto Kinoshita, 17-1, 3-chome, Nishiogi-kita, Suginami-ku, Tokyo; secretary-general

MADAGASCAR: Dr. Rémy Rabary

MALAYSIA: Dr. Siow Keng Ngoh, 545 Serangoon Road, Singapore; director of the Chinese Acupuncture and Cauterization Centre

NORTH VIETNAM: Dr. Nguyen Van Huong; director of the Hanoi Institute of Oriental Medicine

POLAND: Dr. Kobos, Ryszard Nowotki 20 a.m., Warsaw 43

REPUBLIC OF KOREA: Dr. Chang Bin Lee, 18 Don-Ui-Dong-Chong-No-Ku, Seoul; president of the Academic Society of Acupuncture and Moxibustion

Drs. Jin Chang Choe and Jung Kyu Lee, 242 Bokwang-Dong-Yongsan-Ku, Seoul; director and vice-president of the Oriental Medicine Association

ROMANIA: Professor Gheorgiu, Bd. Docia 25 A, Sector II, Bucharest; president of the Bucharest Acupuncture Association

SWITZERLAND: Dr. Guido Fisch, chemin de Mornex 8, Lausanne 1000; president of the Swiss Acupuncture Association

TAIWAN: Dr. Wu Wei Ping, 33 Kiang Ting Road, Taipei; president of the Chinese Acupuncture Association

UNITED KINGDOM: Dr. Rose-Neil, Tyringham, Newport Pagnel, Buckinghamshire

Dr. Felix Mann, 57A Wimpole Street, London, W. 1.; president of the British Acupuncture Association

URUGUAY: Dr. A. Rubens Hermida Barreira, Médico Miguelette 1911, Montevideo; president of the Uruguayan Acupuncture Association

USSR: Professor Tycostchinskaja, Leningrad; director of the Psycho-Neurological Institute

WEST GERMANY: Dr. Schmidt, Neckerstrasse 48B, Stuttgart 7; president of the German Acupuncture Association

APPENDIX F

Recommended Reading in Western Languages

IN ENGLISH

Wu, Wei-ping. *Chinese Acupuncture*. Rustington, Sussex, England, Health Science Press

Veith, Ilza (trans.). *The Yellow Emperor's Classic of Internal Medicine*. Berkeley and Los Angeles, University of California Press

IN FRENCH

Chamfrault, A. *Traité de médecine chinoise*. Angoulême, Editions Coquemard

Morant, Soulié de. *L'Acuponcture chinoise* (5 vols.). Paris, Jacques Lafitte

Niboyet, J. E. H. *Essai sur l'acuponcture chinoise practique*. Paris, Editions Dominique Wapler

IN ITALIAN

Lanza, Uldérico. *Agopunctura e reflessologia*. Turin, privately published

IN SPANISH

Sussman, J. *Acupunctura teoria y practica*. Buenos Aires, Editiones Macchi

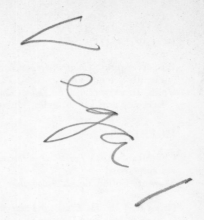 The "weathermark" identifies this book as a production of John Weatherhill, Inc., publishers of fine books on Asia and the Pacific. Supervising editor: Suzanne Trumbull. Book design, typography, and layout of illustrations: Dana Levy. Production supervisor: Mitsuo Okado. Composition: General Printing Company, Yokohama. Offset platemaking and printing: Kinmei Printing Company, Tokyo. Binding: Makoto Binderies, Tokyo. The typeface used is monotype Baskerville, with hand-set Bulmer for display.